DIABETIC KETO COOKBOOK:

The Perfect Step-By-Step Guide For The Preparation Of Simple And Healthy Ketogenic Recipes To Manage Diabetes. Improve Your Meal Plan Today!

Melinda James

© Copyright 2020 - All rights reserved.

The content contained within this book may not be reproduced, duplicated or transmitted without direct written permission from the author or the publisher. Under no circumstances will any blame or legal responsibility be held against the publisher, or author, for any damages, reparation, or monetary loss due to the information contained within this book. Either directly or indirectly.

Legal Notice:

This book is copyright protected. This book is only for personal use. You cannot amend, distribute, sell, use, quote or paraphrase any part, or the content within this book, without the consent of the author or publisher.

Disclaimer Notice:

Please note the information contained within this document is for educational and entertainment purposes only. All effort has been executed to present accurate, up to date, and reliable, complete information. No warranties of any kind are declared or implied. Readers acknowledge that the author is not engaging in the rendering of legal, financial, medical or professional advice. The content within this book has been derived from various sources. Please consult a licensed professional before attempting any techniques outlined in this book.

By reading this document, the reader agrees that under no circumstances is the author responsible for any losses, direct or indirect, which are incurred as a result of the use of information contained within this document, including, but not limited to, errors, omissions, or inaccuracies.

TABLE OF CONTENTS

INTRODUCTION 8

CHAPTER 1: WHY DO WE GET DIABETES? 12
- WHAT IS DIABETES? 12
- THE MAJOR 2 TYPES OF DIABETES 13
- LEARNING TO DIAGNOSE DIABETES 17
- THE SYMPTOMS OF DIABETES 19

CHAPTER 2: SUGARS, THE REAL PROBLEM. 20
- WHAT IS THE GLYCEMIC INDEX 20
- THE LIST BELOW SHOWS THE GLYCEMIC INDEX OF VARIOUS FOODS. 20
- DIABETES TYPE 1 DIET 22
- TYPES OF DIETS FOR TYPE 2 DIABETES 23

CHAPTER 3: INSULIN SPIKES AND BLOOD GLUCOSE. 25
- CONTROLLING YOUR BLOOD SUGAR NATURALLY IN 5 EASY STEPS 25

CHAPTER 4: WHY A LOW CARB DIET CAN BE OF GREAT HELP? 27
- CALORIES & CARBOHYDRATES 30
- LOW CARB DIET TO MANAGE DIABETES 31
- WHAT IS THE OPTIMAL CARBOHYDRATE INTAKE? 31
- CHOOSING THE RIGHT CARBS 32

CHAPTER 5: WHY MEAL PREP? 34
- THE COMMON MISTAKES BY MEAL PREPPING BEGINNERS 35
- THE BENEFITS OF THE DIABETES MEAL PREP 36

CHAPTER 6: THE HEALTH BENEFITS OF USING A KETOGENIC DIET 38
- ADVANTAGES OF THE KETO DIET 39
- CAUTION FOR KETO 43

CHAPTER 7: THE TIPS AND TRICKS THAT HELP YOU CONTAIN DIABETES. 45
- TIPS FOR REVERSING DIABETES 45
- TIPS MAINTAINING YOUR PROGRESS 46

CHAPTER 8: SHOPPING LIST 48

CHAPTER 9: BREAKFAST 53
- GRANOLA WITH FRUITS 53
- APPLE & CINNAMON PANCAKE 54
- SPINACH SCRAMBLE 54
- BREAKFAST PARFAIT 55

Asparagus & Cheese Omelet	55
Sausage, Egg & Potatoes	56
Cucumber & Yogurt	57
Yogurt Breakfast Pudding	57
Vegetable Omelet	58
Almond & Berry Smoothie	59
Easy Veggie Muffins	59
Carrot Muffins	60
Pineapple Oatmeal	61
Spinach Muffins	61
Chia Seeds Breakfast Mix	62
Breakfast Fruits Bowls	62
Pumpkin Breakfast Cookies	63
Veggie Scramble	63
Quinoa Bowls	64
Delicious Yogurt and Fruits	64
Easy Breakfast Fruit Mix	65
Breakfast Apples Mix	65
Veggie Quiche	66
Potato Hash	67
Leeks and Eggs Muffins	67

CHAPTER 10: LUNCH RECIPES 69

Pork Chops with Grape Sauce	69
Roasted Pork & Apples	70
Pork with Cranberry Relish	71
Irish Pork Roast	71
Sesame Pork with Mustard Sauce	72
Steak with Mushroom Sauce	73
Steak with Tomato & Herbs	74
Barbecue Beef Brisket	75
Beef & Asparagus	75

CHAPTER 11: DINNER RECIPES 77

Almond-Crusted Salmon	77
Chicken & Veggie Bowl with Brown Rice	77
Beef Fajitas	79
Sautéed Turkey Bowl	79
Chicken Mushroom Stroganoff	80
Grilled Tuna Kebabs	81
Cast-Iron Pork Loin	82
Crispy Baked Tofu	82
Tilapia with Coconut Rice	83
Spicy Turkey Tacos	84
Quick and Easy Shrimp Stir-Fry	84
Chicken Burrito Bowl with Quinoa	85
Baked Salmon Cakes	86

CHAPTER 12: VEGETABLES 88

    Arugula and Chorizo Salad Recipe 88
    Avocado n Egg Salad 88
    Broccoli Stew with lemon flavor 89
    Brussels Sprouts Soup with chicken stock 90
    Buttered Asparagus 90
    Butternut Squash Salad 91
    Cabbage and Brussels Sprouts Salad 91
    Cabbage with Coconut aminos Salad 92
    Capers Eggplant Medley 92
    Swiss Vegetable Soup 93

CHAPTER 13: MEAT RECIPES 95

    Pork Chops with Grape Sauce 95
    Roasted Pork & Apples 96
    Pork with Cranberry Relish 96
    Irish Pork Roast 97
    Sesame Pork with Mustard Sauce 98
    Steak with Mushroom Sauce 99
    Steak with Tomato & Herbs 99
    Barbecue Beef Brisket 100
    Beef & Asparagus 101

CHAPTER 14: SNACKS 102

    Cinnamon Spiced Popcorn 102
    Grilled Peaches 102
    Peanut Butter Banana "Ice Cream" 103
    Fruity Coconut Energy Balls 103
    Strawberry Salsa 104
    Garden Wraps 104
    Stuffed Moroccan Mushrooms 105
    Party Shrimp 106
    Zucchini Mini Pizzas 107
    Garlic-Sesame Pumpkin Seeds 107
    Roasted Eggplant Spread 108
    Marinated Shrimp 109

CHAPTER 15: DESSERT RECIPES 110

    Chocolate Pudding 110
    Coffee Cream 110
    Walnut Balls 111
    Vanilla Cream 111
    Berry Cream 111
    Cream Cheese Ramekins 112
    Avocado Cream 112
    Strawberry Stew 113

Coconut Muffins	113
Blueberries Mousse	113
Almond Berries Mix	114
Lime and Watermelon Mousse	114
Eggs Cream	115
Chia Squares	115
Plums Stew	115
Plum Cream	116
Cold Berries and Plums Bowls	116
Lime Avocado and Strawberries Mix	117
Avocado and Watermelon Salad	117
Coconut Raspberries Mix	117
Cinnamon Cream	118
Chocolate Cookies	118
Special Dessert	119
Coconut and Mint Cookies	119
Avocado Bars	119
Orange Cake	120
Tasty Nutella	121
Mug Cake	121
Delicious Sweet Buns	122
Lemon Custard	122
CONCLUSION	**123**

Introduction

While many individuals may live with diabetes, there is a great deal that is unknown to those who have it and even more unknown to those who do not. Diabetes is a condition that can affect any individual, from children to the elderly, which is why it is important for all individuals to understand what this condition is, how it can be prevented, and what to do if you are at a higher risk of developing it. Type 2 diabetes can be prevented if one understands its causes and risk factors. We will focus on giving you an understanding of what diabetes is, why glucose and insulin levels become too high or too low, the first signs of type 2 diabetes and how the long-term effects of this condition can put you at risk.

Eating lots of sugar is not the only or even the main cause of diabetes. It also depends on your genetic mutations, family heredity, health, ethnicity, damage to your pancreas, various medications, other diseases, hormonal imbalance and environmental factors. For example, as a rule cystic fibrosis creates a thick excretion (mucus) that can cause scarring in the pancreas. This scarring can keep the pancreas from producing sufficient insulin, leading to diabetes.

Another disease, hemochromatosis, causes the body to store excessive iron. If this disease is not treated in time, it leads to damage of the pancreas, among other organs, and causes diabetes. Diabetes can also be inherited through genes passed along in families, which cause the pancreas to produce less insulin.

Some hormone imbalance conditions such as hyperthyroidism, cause the body to produce too much of the thyroid hormone which can lead to insulin resistance and diabetes. Sometimes diabetes is caused by damage to or removal of the pancreas. This reduces or eliminates the number of insulins producing cells, leading to diabetes.

Certain medications or drugs such as anti-seizure drugs, psychiatric drugs, HIV medications, glucocorticoids, niacin, pentamidine, and diuretics can lead to diabetes because these drugs harm beta cells in the pancreas which produce insulin.

Diabetes leads to certain major health problems like stroke, heart attacks, kidney, dental, eye, nerve, and foot problems.

Heart diseases and strokes: Due to diabetes, blood vessels may be damaged which can lead to some heart diseases and also strokes. You can prevent and avoid strokes and heart diseases by properly maintaining your blood pressure, blood glucose and cholesterol levels, and by avoiding smoking.

Hypoglycemia (low blood glucose): Hypoglycemia strikes suddenly when your blood glucose drops too low. This can be prevented by following a proper diet and meal plan, by medications and by balancing physical activities such as walking.

Diabetic neuropathy (nerve damage): Sometimes nerve damage is also caused by diabetes. Most often the nerve damage will be in the feet, limbs and heart. You can feel when your feet become numb for a long time, in which case you must consult your doctor, because, due to decreased blood flow, this can lead to infection and paralysis.

Kidney problems: Kidney problems caused by diabetes are also known as diabetic nephropathy. If diabetes is poorly controlled, it may lead to kidney failure.

Eye problems: Sometimes poorly controlled diabetes will cause nerve damage in the eyes which may lead to temporary blindness, low vision and even permanent blindness. This can be prevented by managing your blood pressure, blood glucose levels, and regular eye checkups.

Urological and sexual problems: The most common disturbance with diabetes is bladder problems like frequent urination, a burning sensation while urinating, and other complications.

You must be aware of your health.

Most of those who have encountered an unpleasant disease, such as diabetes mellitus (DM) know that this diagnosis means a review of the whole lifestyle. First of all, eating habits should be scrutinized. Unfortunately, there is Sadly, there are no miraculous tablet to solve the problem, so the best course of action is to follow a specific diet, that make it so a diabetic person can eat as they please and pay no mind to sugar levels.

Why Diet for Diabetes

Many books have been written about diabetes, but many fail to mention that proper nutrition is a key aspect of treatment of the disease. After all, diabetes is an endocrine disease that is directly related to one of the essential hormones in the body, insulin. Insulin is produced in the pancreas and is necessary for the absorption of glucose through the digestive tract.

All food consists of three main components: proteins, fats, and carbohydrates. All of these components play an essential role, but carbohydrates (sugars) are of particular importance. Carbohydrates are the primary source of energy for the cells of the human body. More specifically, only one substance performs this function, glucose, which belongs to the class of monosaccharides. Other types of simple carbohydrates are converted to glucose in one way or another. Similar carbohydrates include fructose, sucrose, maltose, lactose, and starch. Finally, some polysaccharides are not absorbed in the digestive tract, like pectin, cellulose, hemicellulose, gum, and dextrin.

Glucose can only independently penetrate neurons, or brain cells. In all other cases, glucose requires a kind of "key." This is insulin. Insulin is a protein that binds to specific receptors on the cell walls, making glucose able to perform its function.

The root cause of diabetes is a failure of this mechanism. In type 1 diabetes, there is an absolute lack of insulin. This means that glucose is missing the "key" and cannot penetrate the cells. The cause of this condition is usually pancreatic disease, as a result of which insulin synthesis drops significantly or even to zero.

In type 2 diabetes, the body still produces insulin. Thus, glucose has a "key" that allows it to enter cells. However, it cannot do this because the "lock" is faulty, meaning the cells do not contain specific protein receptors that are susceptible to insulin. This condition usually develops gradually and has several causes, ranging from excess fat in the body to a genetic predisposition. With the development of the disease, the body may begin to stop producing insulin.

Both conditions are incredibly taxing on the body. Firstly, the glucose that didn't enter the cells begins to accumulate in the blood and is deposited in various tissues, damaging them. Secondly, the body starts to lack the energy that it should have received from glucose.

How can diet help in both of these cases? A healthy diet, avoiding certain inflammatory foods and incorporating others, is intended to supplement the medical treatment of diabetes, and correct metabolic disorders.

As an increased glucose concentration inevitably leads to severe damage to various organs, a proper diet will help stabilize blood glucose levels. Diabetes negatively affects blood vessels, blood circulation worsens, and immunity is reduced. Severe complications are possible: heart attacks, strokes, gangrene.

Treatment of type 1 diabetes should be aimed at stabilizing the level of carbohydrates in the blood. With this type of diabetes, the patient is forced to use injectable insulin, thus the number of carbohydrates supplied by food should correspond to the amount of glucose that insulin can manage. Otherwise, if there is too much or too little insulin, both hyperglycemic (associated with high glucose) and hypoglycemic (associated with low glucose) conditions are possible. Moreover, hypoglycemia in diabetes mellitus, is even more dangerous than hyperglycemia. After all, glucose is the only source of energy for the brain, and its lack of blood can lead to complications such as hypoglycemic coma.

If you are diagnosed with diabetes mellitus, this diet should be followed for the rest of your life to manage symptoms, as there are no complete cures for the disease. However, this does not mean that you will be forever deprived of the pleasure of enjoying your favorite foods. Proper nutrition, along with taking sugar-lowering medicines and insulin, will help stabilize the course of the disease, and in this case, a person can afford some liberties in the diet. Thus, drug treatment and nutrition, contributing to the normalization of carbohydrate metabolism, are the cornerstones of antidiabetic therapy. Of course, treatment with folk remedies is also possible, but only with the supervision and recommendation of the attending physician.

CHAPTER 1:

Why Do We Get Diabetes?

What is Diabetes?

To fully understand the concept of Diabetes, it is important that you have a good understanding of how your body utilizes glucose and insulin and understand what they actually are.

So, let's first start with glucose.

Glucose is a form of sugar and is, generally speaking, the main source of energy, or "fuel" for our body. Whenever the body needs the energy to perform its day to day activities, it starts to burn glucose in order to get the required energy. Glucose is formed in our body whenever the food that we eat gets broken down into various chemicals during digestion. Glucose travels through the bloodstream and enters the cells in our body with the help of insulin. Unlike Glucose though, Insulin is a type of hormone created in the pancreases. Simply put, it acts as a "Key" that allows cells to "open" up a pathway so that glucose can enter and provide the required energy.

Diabetes develops in the body whenever an insulin imbalance is created in the body. Or more specifically, when insulin runs in short supply/or is absent in our body.

When this happens, glucose is unable to enter the cells and as a result, more and more glucose stays in the bloodstream, which leads to the development of the condition known as Diabetes.

To be a bit more scientific, Diabetes is a disease that usually occurs the level of glucose in our blood (also known as blood sugar), spikes up to abnormal levels.

If Diabetes is not properly treated early on, then the blood glucose levels keep on rising, which leads to various health problems, including but not limited to blindness, kidney failure, limb amputation, nerve damage and so on.

While at present, there is no exact cure for Diabetes, it is still very much possible to lead a healthy and normal life with proper management and by eating the right kind of food.

The major 2 types of Diabetes

Currently, the well-established records indicate that there are two types of Diabetes, namely Type 2 and Type 1.

It should be noted that the Type 1 Diabetes was once known as Insulin Dependent Diabetes Mellitus or IDDM or even Juvenile-Onset Diabetes Mellitus. So, if you see any of those two words, don't be alarmed.

I will go into details for both types of Diabetes, however, to give you an overview.

When a person encounters Type- 1 Diabetes, the pancreas starts to experience an autoimmune attack where the body starts to harm itself, making the pancreas incapable of producing the ever so important hormone called "Insulin".

Studies have found a good number of anomalous antibodies in almost all patients suffering from Type – 1 Diabetes.

And just for your information, Antibodies are proteins in your bloodstream that help with the body's immune system.

Therefore, when a person suffers from Type – 1 Diabetes, he/she needs to rely on external medication to get the required amount of insulin.

That being said, now let's have a deeper look into the two different types of Diabetes.

First,

Type – 1

I have already given a brief about Type- 1 Diabetes above, so let's get into the technical details here.

Autoimmune diseases such as Type – 1 Diabetes cause the immune system of our body to accidentally produce anomalous inflammatory cells and antibodies that, instead of protecting the body, try to damage the healthy cells of the patient's body.

For Type -1, the beta cells found in the pancreas, which are specifically responsible for producing insulin, get attacked by these anomalous antibodies.

It is largely believed all around that the tendency to actually develop anomalous antibodies during Type -1 is inherited genetically. Though, the studies on this topic are still ongoing and not concrete.

It has been seen that exposure to various viral infections such as Coxsackie Virus or Mumps or various other environmental toxins might also be responsible to trigger the production of anomalous antibodies that might ultimately go and damage the beta cells of the pancreas.

Some of the most common antibodies seen in patients of Type-1 Diabetes include

- Anti-Glutamic Decarboxylase
- Anti-Insulin
- Anti-Islet

Currently, the American Diabetes Association does not really recommend a general screening for individuals suffering from Type -1 Diabetes, however, individuals people who are seemingly at high risks, such as those having a first degree relative (such a parent or sibling) with diagnosed diabetes are highly encouraged to have themselves screened.

Recent studies have shown that Type-1 diabetes is more common in young ones, usually under the age of 30. However, older patients have also been seen to get affected by Type – 1.

The individuals who develop Diabetes at a very late stage of life fall into a subcategory of people who are said to have LADA or Latent Autoimmune Diabetes in Adults.

This basically means that they actually had diabetes from an early stage, but for some reason, it remained latent in their body.

LADA is very slow and, in a way, progressive form of Diabetes (Type -1).

All in all, though, currently only about 10% of the whole population suffering from diabetes tend to have Type 1, while the other 90% suffer from Type 2.

Type – 2

Non-Insulin Dependent Diabetes Mellitus (NIDDM) or even Adult- Onset Diabetes Mellitus are two of the scientific name that was previously used to describe Type-2 Diabetes.

A patient suffering from Type -2 Diabetes will still be able to produce insulin as the production does not completely come to a halt, however, the amount of insulin produced is significantly lower than the minimum amount requires by the body to stay healthy.

In some cases, though, the exact opposite might happen, resulting in the production of a large amount of insulin than that is required by the body!

One of the major caveats of Type-2 is that it basically makes the cells of the body particularly insensitive to insulin.

But that's not all, in addition to the problem mentioned above, the pancreas develops a form of insulin resistance that defects the release of insulin by the pancreas.

In fact, it has already been seen that a very steady decline of beta-cell insulin production happens in Type -1 that leads to even worse control of glucose in the bloodstream.

This is also one of the main reasons why patients with Type -2 Diabetes tend to undergo insulin therapy in the long run.

And lastly, the liver of patients suffering from Type-1 also starts to undergo Gluconeogenesis despite the already above normal levels of glucose in the bloodstream, which ultimately causes the liver to flood the bloodstream with even more glucose.

It is mostly believed that Type-2 primarily affects individuals who are over 30 years old, however, that's not necessarily true. While it is true that the possibility of getting the effect with Type-2 does increase with age, it is still seen that more and more teenagers are starting to develop Type-2 at a very early age.

Most of these cases are due to a lack of regular exercise, having higher than normal body weight, abnormal eating habits and so on.

Just as before, Genetic inheritance is also a major risk factor of Type 2, however, there are some others that you should be aware of as well. And the most significant one out of them is "Obesity". It has been seen that there is a very strong and direct relationship between the degree of obesity that a person is suffering from and the risk of developing Type-2.

And perhaps the worst part is that this is true for both young ones as well as adults. In fact, it has been estimated that the possibility of developing diabetes almost doubles for about a 20% increase over a body's normal desired weight.

As for age, data shows that for every 10 years in the crease after the age of 40, regardless of an individual's weight, the possibility of suffering from diabetes increases significantly.

The prevalence of diabetes is about 25% in individuals 65 years or older.

It has also been seen that the possibility of suffering from Type-2 varies from one ethnic group to the other as well.

For example, the prevalence rate is 7% In Non-Hispanic Caucasians while it is 8% in Asian Americans, 13% in Hispanics, 12.3% in Blacks and 20-50% in Native Americans.

The other types to know about

Apart from the ones mentioned above, there are some other types of diabetes that you should be aware of.

Secondary Diabetes

This type of diabetes refers to an abnormally elevated level of blood sugar happening from any other form of medical medication.

Secondary Diabetes might develop when an individual is suffering from pancreatic issues that may destroy the capacity of the pancreas to produce insulin. A quick example would be chronic pancreatitis.

Just in case you don't know, chronic pancreatitis essentially is the inflammation of your pancreas caused by toxins due to excess alcoholism. Other than that, surgical removal pancreas or certain types of trauma might also result in this.

Gestational Diabetes

It should be noted that Diabetes can actually happen for a temporary period of time during pregnancy. And in fact, it has been suggested that almost 2-10% of all pregnancies result in temporary diabetes. During pregnancy, a great deal of hormonal changes takes place that might lead to a spike in blood sugar levels. Gestational Diabetes refers to this scenario when the blood sugar level elevates to abnormal levels during pregnancy due to hormonal changes. It does not last long though as Gestational Diabetes usually goes away after the birthing is complete. Unfortunately, though, almost 35% - 60% of the women who suffer from gestational diabetes usually tend to develop type -2 after about 10-20 years of pregnancy. This is truer for individuals who required the injection of external insulin during pregnancy or those who fail to maintain their weight after delivery. Women who are suspected to have gestational diabetes often are encouraged to take an oral glucose tolerance test around six weeks after delivery to ensure keep their diabetes in check and know if their gestational diabetes is developing into something more.

Hormonal Disturbances

Apart from that, Diabetes can also come from various types of hormonal disturbances. Excessive production of growth hormones alongside Cushing's syndrome might lead to diabetes.

In acromegaly (excess growth hormone production), the pituitary gland tends to cause excessive production of growth hormone that leads to hyperglycemia.

In Cushing's syndrome, on the other hand, the adrenal gland tends to lose control and produce a large amount of another hormone known as "Cortisol" that leads to increase blood sugar elevation as well.

Medication-related Diabetes

Apart from all of the scenarios mentioned above, you should know that Diabetes can also occur from various kinds of medications that might make your body to lose control of your diabetes or provoke latent diabetes to surface up.

Individuals who mostly take medications such as steroids or are taking medications to treat HIV are more at risk of developing diabetes.

Learning to diagnose diabetes

Diagnosing if you have diabetes or not is actually easier than most people think. At present, there are two leading methods of diagnosing diabetes at home, which is testing your blood or an oral glucose test.

I will be talking a bit about both here.

First, let's talk about the blood glucose test.

Blood Glucose Test

So, when testing your blood glucose, a method called the "Fasting Blood Glucose" method is generally followed and is the preferred way to diagnose diabetes. It is extremely simple to do and convenient. The core instruction here is to simply fast overnight (or for at least 8 hours), take a small sample of blood and analyze the blood.

This can be done easily at home using various portable devices, or you can visit a doctor or diagnostics lab to have it checked.

If you are doing at home, what you must understand is:

- Normal levels for plasma glucose should be less than 100 mg/dl
- Glucose levels more than 126 mg/dl on more than two different occasions indicate diabetes
- And lastly, a random test (without fasting) that gives a count of 200 mg/dl or more indicates diabetes too.

Oral Glucose Tolerance Test

This method is not really used routinely these days, but the OGTT is pretty much the best when it comes to diagnosing Type-2 Diabetes.

It is still regularly used for checking individuals with symptoms of gestational diabetes.

For the Oral Test, a person is required to fast overnight (at least 8 or a maximum of 16 hours).

Once that is done, the first step is to check the person for the fasting glucose.

Once that, the person is given an oral dose (about 75gm) or glucose. After which, the blood is taken at several intervals.

Keep in mind that there are various other methods deployed by obstetricians, but the one mentioned above is considered to be the standard one.

There are certain steps that one should take though before taking the test, those are:

- It is essential that the person is in good health
- It is essential that the person is active
- It should be checked that the person is not taking any medicine that might affect the blood glucose levels
- On the day of the test, the individual should not indulge in any form of drinking or smoking, not even coffee.

The original version of the Oral Test used to measure the level of blood glucose 5 times over a long session of 3 hours.

Some physicians, on the other hand, tend to get a baseline sample that is followed by just another sample about 2 hours after from the time of drinking the glucose drink.

For an individual who has no diabetes, the level of glucose will immediately spike after the drink and then drop rapidly.

For people with diabetes, the levels will rise up to an abnormal level and stay there.

To summarize the results:

- If a person has a glucose level that is less than 140mg/dl after 2 hours from taking the glucose solution, with the level less than 200 mg/dl during the 2 hours the person is said to have a normal response.

- If a person has a glucose level that is less than 126mg/dl after 2 hours from taking the glucose solution, with the level hovering around 140-199 mg/dl during the 2 hours, the person is said to have an impaired glucose tolerance.
- If two diagnostics tests done on two different days shows a high glucose result, then the person has diabetes
- In the case of pregnant women, a fasting glucose level of 92 mg/dl, after an hour a level of 180 mg/dl and after 2 hours a level of 153 mg/dl would dictate that the women have gestational diabetes.

The symptoms of Diabetes

Checking your blood or having an oral test aren't the only two ways how you can check your Diabetes. There are certain signs and symptoms that you should keep an eye out for, that might imply that you have Diabetes.

The most common ones are:

For Type 1:

- Patches of dark skin, round neck or armpits
- Being frequently affected by infection
- Delayed healing of sores
- Having a blurry vision
- Constant fatigue
- Unwanted loss of weight
- Constantly increased hunger
- Increase urination
- Constant sensation of thirst

For Type 2:

- Unwanted weight loss
- Numbness or sensation of pain in feet/hand
- Bruises might take longer to heal
- The extreme level of fatigue
- Increase urination
- The feeling of constant hunger
- Blurred vision

CHAPTER 2:

Sugars, The Real Problem.

What is the glycemic index

In many diabetic diets, the concept of the glycemic index (GI) is widely used. This term refers to the ability of products to cause an increase in blood glucose. This indicator is not equivalent to such parameters as carbohydrate and calorie content. The higher the glycemic index, then the higher the glucose level. As a rule, when there is an equal amount of carbohydrates in several products, GI is higher in those where the proportion of simple sugars is higher, and the content of plant fibers is lower. A GI of less than 40 is considered low, between 40 and 70 is considered average, and an index of more than 70 is considered high. It is especially important for patients with insulin-dependent diabetes mellitus or severe cases of type 2 diabetes to know the GI of food they consume. Therefore, GI can be used to compile an optimal diet.

The list below shows the glycemic index of various foods.

Name	GI	Name	GI	Name	GI
Apricots	35	Grapefruit	25	Rice porridge	70
Cherry plum	25	Fresh mushrooms	10	Gooseberry	40
Pineapples	65	Pears	33	Boiled corn	70
Oranges	40	Melons	45	Cornflakes	85
Fresh Peanuts	15	Potato casserole	90	Dried apricots	30

Watermelons	70	Greenery	0-15	Pasta	60
Eggplant	10	Wild strawberry	40	Raspberry	30
Bananas	60	Marshmallows	80	Mango	55
Sweet potato	74	Raisins	65	Tangerines	40
White loaf	80	Squash and eggplant caviar	15	Honey	80
Black beans	80	Figs	35	Milk, 6%	30
Waffles	76	Natural yogurt	35	Raw carrots	35
Rice Vermicelli	58	Zucchini	15	Boiled carrots	85
Grape	40	Cocoa with milk	40	Cucumbers	25
Cherry	25	White cabbage and cauliflower	15	Walnuts	15
Glucose	100	Broccoli	10	Pizza	60
Blueberry	55	Fried potato	95	Sausages	28
Green peas	35	Boiled potatoes	70	Pumpkin	75
Garnet	30	Oatmeal porridge	40	Dates	103

Diabetes Type 1 Diet

Properly selected nutrition for type 1 diabetes is no less important than the use of insulin-containing drugs.

Currently, doctors believe that with diseases associated with the constant use of insulin, it is not necessary to strictly limit the intake of carbohydrates, as this can lead to hypoglycemic comas and impaired glucose tolerance.

Nevertheless, the patient needs to keep a record of their daily carbohydrates consumed. To simplify this task, diabetologists have proposed a particular unit for measuring the number of carbohydrates in food: the bread. The bread unit is the number of sugars contained in 25g of bread, or about half a slice cut from a loaf. As for other carbohydrates, the bread corresponds to approximately 12g of sugar. The intensity of processing a single bread unit with insulin varies depending on the time of day. More insulin (2 units) is required in the morning, less (1.5 units) in the afternoon, and the least (1 unit) in the evening.

What can I eat with insulin-dependent diabetes without severe restrictions? This list includes foods that contain a meager amount of carbohydrates. First of all, these carbohydrate sources are vegetables that do not contain the bread unit.

- ✔ cucumbers
- ✔ squash
- ✔ zucchini
- ✔ greens (sorrel, spinach, lettuce, chives)
- ✔ mushrooms
- ✔ tomatoes
- ✔ radish
- ✔ pepper
- ✔ cabbage (cauliflower and white)

Sugar-laden drinks, sweet tea, lemonade, and juices are strictly prohibited. After waking, a small snack is needed before insulin is injected to avoid a sharp drop in blood sugar.

Type 1 diabetes is a dangerous disease that can threaten with serious complications like hypoglycemic crisis. This occurs when there is an excess of insulin and a lack of glucose. Therefore, it is recommended to measure the level of glucose in the blood several times a day, every day. If the level has dropped too low (below 4 mmol/L), then you need to take a glucose tablet.

Features of nutrition for type 2 diabetes

Type 2 diabetes develops gradually, and therefore patients are generally not threatened with hyperglycemia and hypoglycemic crisis due to errors in the diet. However, this does not mean that with type 2 diabetes the patient can eat whatever he or she wants. The nutritional model for type 2 diabetes mellitus should be no less strict than for insulin-dependent diabetes. However, periodic deviations from the norm are allowed and do not threaten serious consequences. The main principle of the diet is to restrict the intake of carbohydrates, primarily simple ones. In most cases, the menu for type 2 diabetes mellitus should be combined with the use of sugar-lowering drugs, and in severe stages of the disease, the introduction of insulin.

In treating diabetes, it is necessary to adhere to the proper diet and maintain a healthy body weight. In the diet formulated for those with type 1 diabetes, calories are not reduced, and in the diet for those with type 2, calories are reduced.

Immediate results should not be expected from a change in diet. As a rule, the onset of the therapeutic effect begins after a week, or even months for some.

The main thing is to adhere to proper nutrition. I believe in you!

Types of diets for type 2 diabetes

Dietitians have gained extensive experience in treating diabetes with proper nutrition. However, the exact prescriptions are often different in some details. Therefore, there are many different diets that cater to different needs.

The main varieties of diets:

- low carbohydrate diet
- carbohydrate-free diet
- high protein diet
- buckwheat diet
- vegetarian diet
- table number 9
- American Diabetes Association Diet

This list of diets is primarily designed for non-insulin-dependent diabetes. Their use in insulin-dependent diabetes is also still possible. Each of them has advantages and disadvantages.

As for popular fasting techniques, most nutritional schools find no beneficial effects for those with diabetes.

What diet should you followed? Choosing the best diet does not need to be done alone, but with the help of an experienced specialist, an endocrinologist. It is essential to choose a diet that the patient will not only be able to adhere to, but also enjoy. Otherwise, it is likely that the diet will not be followed, and all efforts to treat the disease will go down the drain.

CHAPTER 3:

Insulin Spikes and Blood Glucose.

When a spike in blood glucose levels occurs, the most common way to lower it down fast is by administering insulin injections. This is something that is simply done every time blood glucose level rises. Dosage and administration should be prescribed by the doctor. There should be adequate knowledge about frequency of injection, how much insulin to use and how often should corrective doses be given.

What's the fastest way to lower blood sugar levels fast naturally?

A spike in blood sugar levels can make a person feel extremely sleepy, cranky and fatigued or experience a feeling of increased thirst. When this happens, the fastest way to lower the blood sugar is to simply exercise or engage in a low to medium-impact physical activity. Exercise helps increase one's sensitivity to insulin. When you exercise, the muscle cells consume the glucose so there will be less of it circulating in the bloodstream.

Following a regular exercise routine is very important when it comes to controlling glucose levels in the blood. It prevents diabetes-related complications such as heart and kidney diseases. However, if you are suffering from type 1 diabetes, it is important to check for urine ketones before exercising, particularly if the glucose level is 250 mg/dl. Exercise is not recommended if ketones are present.

Controlling Your Blood Sugar Naturally In 5 Easy Steps

Now that you are armed with information about diabetes, it's time to put the reversal plan into action. Controlling blood sugar levels will not be easy. The hardest battle would be fighting the feeling of ravenous hunger that diabetics mostly experience. However, with the right strategy, reducing or completely eliminating dependence on insulin or oral drugs is possible.

Step 1 - The first thing that you need to do is to clear the kitchen of all the things that can spike up blood glucose levels, particularly refined sugar and regular table salt. This also includes chips, pastries, chocolates, candies, etc. This is to remove any temptation that can ruin the diabetes reversal efforts.

Step 2 - Prep your food choices for the following 30 days. This program does not impose a strict day-by-day meal plan. Instead, it requires you to put together a diabetic-friendly cookbook. This gives you freedom to choose the meals you want to eat for the day. The idea is to hone you to become a responsible eater.

Step 3 - Head to the grocery and buy your essentials. This includes acceptable sweeteners (e.g. stevia, Xylitol, brown rice syrup) and salt substitutes (e.g. vegetable seasoning). Include the ingredients you plan to cook for the week. Take time to do grocery shopping at the start of each week so you will be stocked up and armed to cook your meals based on your recipe collection.

Step 4 - Plan your exercise regimen. Aerobic conditioning exercise is the best prescribed treatment for diabetes. Choose an exercise that is most convenient for you. These can include jogging, swimming, cycling, treadmill, and other activities that will keep the heart rate sustained for at least 20 minutes. The activity should be done at least 4 times a week. You can also alternate activities such as going swimming during the weekends and jogging and treadmill during weekdays.

Step 5 - Learn to cook your own foods. If you're not the type of person who cooks, then this is the best time to learn. Taking control of your food is the key to preventing blood sugar levels from spiking up. Food cooked commercially is too risky for diabetics because it contains high levels of sodium, artificial flavors, synthetic seasonings and refined sweeteners. Be prepared to give up some of the dine-in, take-outs or street foods you are used to eating. There are a lot of diabetic-friendly meals that are delicious and appropriate to eat that you will surely get used to.

CHAPTER 4:

Why A Low Carb Diet Can Be Of Great Help?

Some foods will increase blood glucose levels more than others. To manage diabetes, it is important to know what you should eat and how much you must consume. It is essential to follow a healthy eating plan that will fit your lifestyle. This will help you control your blood glucose.

Mainly we have 3 nutrients in food. They are carbohydrates, proteins, and fats.

1. Carbohydrates

Carbs include sugar, starches, and fiber obtained from foods like fruits, grains, milk products, vegetables, and sweets. They will increase the blood glucose levels in your body faster compared to other nutrients, such as fats and proteins.

You must know the foods that have carbs and their quantities in a meal. It is always better that you get carbohydrates from healthy sources, such as fruits, whole grains that are fiber-rich and vegetables. Avoid or limit the intake of carbohydrates from salt, fat, and those with added sugar.

2. Proteins

Proteins are essential in a balanced diet. Apart from giving you key nutrients, they will also prevent you from feeling hungry, so you will not overeat. Proteins won't directly increase the glucose levels like carbohydrates. But you will still need to control the intake of proteins.

Protein will make insulin work faster for those who have type-2 diabetes. So, it is a good idea to also limit the consumption of protein shakes and mixes.

3. Fats

Like proteins, you must also consume fats to have a balanced diet, particularly healthy fats that you will have from nuts, seeds, and fatty fish. Fats won't increase blood glucose levels, but they have a lot of calories, which can cause obesity.

Weight gain is not good because obese people are more likely to suffer from the disease. So, a diabetic diet will contain the consumption of fats.

Carbohydrates are very important in diabetic food. You have to watch out for how much you are eating and must also ensure that they are spread out throughout the day so that your blood glucose level is properly managed.

Usually, a diabetic person will be told to make sure that 40% to 55% of the calorie intake daily is from the carbs. But there can be exceptions. A nutritionist can recommend fewer or more carbs depending on specific health conditions.

However, having said this, the food pyramid of a person with diabetes isn't all that different. The foods on the menu include different types of fruits, vegetables, and grains. Usually, you will be asked to consume,

- 6-11 servings of grains, legumes or bread and starchy vegetables
- 2-4 fruit servings
- 3-5 non-starchy vegetable servings
- 2-3 servings of yogurt or milk products
- 2-3 protein servings from meat substitutes or meat

Food Group	What you can have	Alternative
Fruit (15-gram carbs in 1 serving)	A medium or small fresh fruit	Half cup fresh juice. You can also have chopped or canned fruit. Fresh is always best.
Vegetable (5 grams carbs in each serving)	1 cup of raw vegetables	Half cup of vegetable juice or cooked vegetables

Starch (15 grams carbs in each serving)	1 ounce or slice of bread	Half cup cereal, pasta or starchy vegetables.
Honey, molasses, sugar	1 teaspoon	4 grams of carbohydrates
Milk (without any cheese, yogurt, or cream)	1 cup milk	8 grams of protein and 12 grams of carbs
Meat	1 ounce of yogurt or cheese, poultry, fish, meat	Half cup of dried beans.
Fat (this includes seeds, nuts, little bit of peanut butter and bacon	1 teaspoon of oil, margarine or butter	5 grams of fat

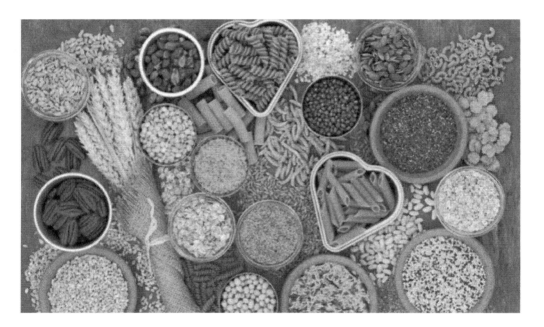

Follow these food rules –

- Eat foods that have healthy fiber and carbohydrates
- Include whole grains, such as oats, quinoa, legumes like beans, fresh non-starchy vegetables, sweet potatoes, and whole fruits.
- You should have heart-healthy omega-3 fatty acids, such as sardines, tuna, salmon, mackerel, cod, halibut, and flax seeds in the food menu.

- Get monounsaturated and polyunsaturated fats from peanut oil, olive oil, canola oil, avocados, and nuts, such as pecans, almonds, and walnuts.
- Read all food labels carefully.
- Also, remember to eat at the right time and not too overeat.
- Spread food throughout the day.
- Avoid the foods that are rich in trans or saturated fats, processed meats, organ meat like beef or liver, margarine, white bread, shellfish, dairy products with a lot of fat, processed snacks, white rice, pasta, and sugary drinks.

Lifestyle and food changes will both have a big effect.

Like food, lifestyle is also very important. These days, so many of us are leading a sedentary lifestyle, and not getting enough exercise. Thanks to our desk jobs and modern cars, we are not even walking that much anymore. Add to that the oily, greasy foods and junk foods with unhealthy ingredients, and it's no surprise that we have a generation full of obese people. It's a global problem. But it is most serious in the western, developed world.

It is a known fact that obesity is a major cause of diabetes, especially type 2. Those who are obese even by a few pounds are at a considerably higher risk.

So, it is essential to count the calories and carbohydrates you are eating. Shed those excess pounds, switch to a healthy diabetic diet, get adequate exercise, and you will be able to reduce the risk immensely. This routine is essential even to manage diabetes if you already have the illness. Even daily brisk walking for an hour, 5 days a week will help. Many experts recommend walking for 250 minutes a week.

It is even better if you can do some jogging or running. Cycling, swimming, and playing a sport is going to be even better. Take the staircase instead of the elevator. Simple steps can make a huge difference.

Calories & Carbohydrates

When you have diabetes, your body will face problems in processing carbohydrates efficiently. So, it is essential to limit the intake of carbs. However, finding out how many carbohydrates to eat can still be confusing.

Many dietary guidelines recommend that diabetic people should have 45% to 60% of their calories daily from carbohydrates. But some experts believe that diabetics should eat even fewer carbs. Some of them in fact, recommend that the percentage of carbs should be half of this.

Low Carb Diet to Manage Diabetes

Several studies have revealed that low-carb diets are good for treating diabetes. In fact, low carbohydrate diets were standard treatments for treating the disease before insulin was discovered in 1921. These diets also seem to work for the long-term as long as you stick to the food regimen.

In this study, the subjects were asked to eat a low carbohydrate diet for six months. It was found that their diabetes stayed within control even 3 years after the study was over, provided the participants followed the recommended food menu.

Not just type-2, a diabetic menu also helps those who are suffering from type-1. Studies have shown that there can be a significant improvement in the blood sugar levels if the recommended diet is followed.

What is the optimal carbohydrate intake?

Though many experts have forwarded their opinion on how much carbohydrates you should have, but there is no unanimity on this, even among those who recommend carb restriction. Several studies have found that there is a big improvement in weight, blood sugar level, and other health markers when the carbohydrate intake is limited to 20 grams daily.

But there are exceptions. For instance, Dr. Richard K. Bernstein, who himself suffers from type-1 diabetes, has found that many of his patients who take 30 grams of carbohydrates every day were able to achieve blood sugar control.

There is also research that shows that a more moderate regimen of 70 to 90 grams of carbs, which means getting 20% of the calories from carbohydrates, may also be effective. Also, the carb amount will vary from one person to another as all of us respond a bit differently to carbohydrates.

ADA or the American Diabetes Association says that there cannot be any one solution for everyone. Customized meal plans, which consider metabolic goals and dietary preferences are thus the best.

But it is generally believed that you can have between 6 and 25 grams of carbs in a meal if your blood sugar is lower than 140 mg/dL (8 mmol/L).

Always remember, as a general rule, your blood sugar will rise less if you take fewer carbs. Also, it is not a good idea to completely eliminate carbs. You should have a healthy low-carb diet full of nutrient-rich, high-fiber carbohydrates, such as berries, seeds, nuts, and vegetables.

Choosing the right Carbs

Carbs you get from fresh vegetables are always good. They are made up of fiber, sugar, and starch. Only the sugar and starch components will increase your blood sugar.

The fiber you get naturally in food, whether it is insoluble or soluble, won't break down into glucose, and it won't increase the blood sugar level. You can even subtract fiber from the carbohydrate, which gives you digestible carb. For instance, 1 cup of cauliflower has 5 grams of carbs, out of which 3 are fiber. So, you get 2 grams of carb.

Prebiotic fiber like insulin can even improve fasting blood sugar, apart from other health markers.

Portion Control

This is very important for people with diabetes. You should stay away from the bad foods as much as possible till the time you have some control over your diabetes. However, this doesn't mean that you cannot ever eat small candy or chocolate.

Portion control means keeping control of the intake of proteins, carbs, dairy products and fats in each serving. Here are some guidelines to follow –

- A baseball or small apple, the size of your clenched fist, is about 1 cup serving or yogurt or fruit

- A deck of cards is about 3 oz. serving of fish, meat, or poultry
- Your thumb tip from the knuckle is the right size of 1 teaspoon of butter or mayonnaise
- A Chapstick tube is the correct size of 1 oz. of cheese

to start with, you may feel like you are not getting enough nutrition, and you may feel like starving, particularly when you see that the others have bigger portion sizes. But remember, you need control over what you consume. In the long-term, you are going to be healthier, which will make you feel better.

Here are some snack substitutes that will prevent you from feeling deprived.

- ½ cup of sugar-free pudding
- 3 cups of air-popped popcorn
- A sugar-free serving of jello
- 20 baked tortilla chips with salsa

CHAPTER 5:

Why Meal Prep?

Whether you are too busy to cook, or you are someone with special dietary requirements, meal prep can help you maintain a healthier lifestyle.

Meal planning also helps you achieve the following:

1. Save time

When you have your meals prepared beforehand, you won't have to spend time thinking about what to eat, do the grocery, and cook food on that day. Instead, you can use the time you save on exercising and other activities that contribute to your well-being.

2. Save money

One of the major benefits of meal prep is the monetary savings. For one, buying in bulk helps you reduce overall food costs. It's also cheaper to cook at home than to eat out, which is what usually happens when you're hungry and have no time for food preparation.

3. Stay on top of your goals

Do you need to watch your carb intake? Or, do you just want to ensure that you're eating nutritionally balanced whole foods? Whatever the reason, meal prepping helps you stay on track and makes achieving your goals much more manageable.

4. Control your portions

Part of meal prep is portion control as it entails planning how much food you have to cook for a certain number of meals. Placing food in individual containers allows for both controlling portions as well as the ease of having food you can easily bring on the go.

5. Manage hunger

Having your food already prepared helps you stave off hunger pangs, so you won't be tempted to eat out or make unwise food choices. For diabetics, having a meal that you can eat whenever you feel hungry is necessary to keep your blood sugar levels normal.

The Common Mistakes by Meal Prepping Beginners

To take advantage of the benefits meal planning has to offer, make sure you avoid the following mistakes:

Mistake # 1 - Not tailoring your meal plan according to your unique needs

It's now very easy to prep meals. You can even download meal plans right to your smartphone or tablet, so you won't have to do the planning yourself. Unfortunately, this could cause some problems especially if you have special dietary requirements. Therefore, before you start making a grocery list, talk to your doctor or a nutritionist who can help you tailor your meal plan based on your specific needs.

For those with diabetes, the American Diabetes Association provides general dietary guidelines on their website, although it is still best that you contact a certified diabetes educator or a registered dietician who can keep track of your individual progress and recommend adjustments, if needed.

Mistake # 2 - Not preparing balanced meals

Whether they are diabetic or not, many people make the mistake of having too much of one or two food groups while neglecting the others. While you can't have too much carbohydrates if you have diabetes or if you're on a certain weight loss plan, carbs are a necessary part of a healthy diet and should be a component of every balanced meal.

On the other hand, just because fats don't have a direct effect on blood glucose levels doesn't mean you can eat too much. Fatty foods can slow down digestion and make it even more difficult for the insulin in your body to do its work. It also increases the risk of cardiovascular problems.

Mistake # 3 - Doing all your meal prep once a week

Weekends are ideal for prepping meals for the whole week. However, if you prepare all your meals for the following six days on Sunday, for example, the meals that you eat towards the end of the week either don't taste good or have already spoiled. This is why it's best to do your meal prep twice: once on the weekend and another in the middle of the week.

Mistake # 4 - Not storing your food properly

Improper storage is another common cause of food spoilage. Thus, it is important to use the appropriate container for each type of food. Where you put your pre-prepared meals is also something to consider.

Make sure to place the food in a refrigerator that is kept below 40 degrees Fahrenheit. Of course, following food safety practices in the food prep area is essential to avoid cross contamination and food poisoning.

The Benefits of the Diabetes Meal Prep

Meal planning is extremely helpful in many practical ways, but one of its greatest benefits is on a person's health, particularly if it combines healthy balanced food and proper portion control.

Benefit # 1 - It helps improve your general health

Whether or not you have a medical condition, meal planning can help you improve your overall health when the meals provide all the macro and micronutrients your body needs. It also helps you avoid saturated fats and processed sugars, which is what most people would reach for if they're hungry and just want something satisfying.

Benefit # 2 - It ensures that you can eat on time

Preparing your meals in advance helps manage hunger pains. Missing a meal or delaying it can cause your blood sugar level to drop too low, a condition otherwise known as hypoglycemia.

Hypoglycemia can cause shaking, disorientation, and irritability. You may even have a seizure if your blood sugar level gets any lower. Having your meal already prepared ensures that you can always eat on time and, therefore, decrease the risk of low blood glucose.

Benefit # 3 - It lowers your risk of heart disease

Diabetes increases the risk of heart disease. With the help of a dietician, planning your meals can help you reduce this risk. Because meal prep reduces the time you need to spend in the kitchen, you'll have more opportunities to exercise and do other activities that promote a healthier lifestyle.

Benefit # 4 - It lowers your risk of cancer

Diabetes also increases the risk of all forms of cancer. While experts are still unable to identify the exact link between these two conditions, they expect that it has something to do with insulin resistance and obesity. Cancer patients are advised to pursue a healthy lifestyle, which includes eating a balanced diet and getting adequate exercise. Because these activities are also encouraged among diabetics, the risk of cancer is lowered.

Benefit # 5 - It helps you maintain healthy body weight

Again, portion control plays a part in this area. Even if you eat healthy food, over-indulging can lead to an unhealthy weight gain, which can make it harder to control your blood sugar level.

If left unchecked, this could lead to high blood sugar levels or hyperglycemia, which can cause various complications that include heart and liver damage as well as loss of kidney function.

It's important to note that while meal planning can help keep the effects of diabetes under control, you and your dietician still need to conduct a periodic review of its effectiveness and make changes whenever necessary.

CHAPTER 6:

The Health Benefits Of Using A Ketogenic Diet

Once you have reached the required level of carbs and maintained for at least a week, your body will burn through its stores of glucose and start activating core ketogenic processes. The liver then breaks down stored fat into a pair of molecules, fatty acid, and glycerol. Fatty acids are what makes it possible for the body to create ketones in the first place, while the glycerol fills in for the glucose in specific instances where the ketones can't provide what the body needs. One such part of the body is the brain as it creates energy through what is known as gluconeogenesis.

While working to literally melt the fat off your body is a great start, there are numerous additional benefits when it comes to remaining in the ketogenic state for a prolonged period of time. What's more, the longer the state persists, the more pronounced the positive effects become. Improves immune system: aside from what it is capable of doing to your overall level of hunger, the ketogenic state is known to dramatically reduce the likelihood of numerous major health issues, starting with all of the types of cancer that are known to feed on glucose directly. While healthy cells can easily switch to burning ketones for energy, cancer cells are not that lucky which means they grow significantly more slowly than they otherwise would when deprived of their primary food source.

Switching to the keto diet is also ideal when it comes to promoting brain health for several reasons. The most important of these is the fact that following the keto diet is closer to the way early humans likely ate which means it is more in line with the type of fuel that the brain is naturally used to consuming. This, in turn, makes it possible for the brain to continue working at maximum capacity for longer than would otherwise be the case.

While it's true that the brain requires glucose to work properly, this is definitely the case of potentially having too much of a good thing. In this instance, if the brain receives too much glucose on a regular basis, then over time it will develop a higher tolerance which means that it will need to work harder in order to generate the same results. If left untreated this can lead to a state of glucose deprivation which can eventually lead to dementia. Utilizing glycerol as a replacement for glucose can then make it easier for the brain to function in the long-term without having to worry about these types of adverse effects, meaning that it is far more likely that degradation will occur. Decreases hunger: beyond simply helping you to burn fat more effectively, following a keto diet is also a great way to lose weight for a number of other reasons, starting with the fact that remaining in ketosis is actually proven to help you to remain feeling full after a meal far longer than would otherwise be the case. This is simply due to the fact that fat is more difficult to process than carbs which means your body won't begin to send out signals saying it is hungry until everything has been completely processed. Additionally, while you can expect some carb cravings during the early part of ketosis, you will find that after you make it past this hurdle you will be able to remove food from your thoughts more easily than before. This is thanks to a useful hormone known as cholecystokinin which is the natural counter to ghrelin, the hormone responsible for telling you when you are hungry. Cholecystokinin is created by the body when food is moving through the intestines, but if you are in ketosis then it will be created at all times instead. The increased cholecystokinin production will continue for the full time your body remains in a ketogenic state, and even for a few days after you have left it. What's more, besides making you look and feel better, the keto diet will also help you to feel fuller, longer and after eating a smaller serving of food. This is a natural side effect of a high fat and protein diet as both of these will stick with you much longer than any type of carbohydrates will. What's more, after you have entered a ketogenic state then your body will naturally start by burning visceral fat which is primarily fat that is stored in the midsection. All in all, a ketogenic state creates a scenario where your chance of heart disease decreases while your level of positive cholesterol increases. It is also known to reduce your risk of stroke and various other cardiovascular issues.

Advantages of the Keto diet

The Keto diet has been proven to have many advantages for people over 50. Here are some of the best.

Strengthens bones

When people get older, their bones weaken. At 50, your bones at likely not as strong as they used to be however, you can keep them in really good conditions. Consuming milk to give calcium cannot do enough to strengthen your bones. What you can do, is to make use of the Keto diet as it is low in toxins. Toxins negatively affect the absorption of nutrients and so with this, your bones can take in all they need.

Eradicates inflammation

Few things are worse than the pain from an inflamed joint or muscle. Arthritis, for instance, can be extremely hard to bear. When you use the ketosis diet, the production of cytokines would be reduced. Cytokines inflammation and so, their eradication would reduce it.

It eradicates nutrients deficiency

Keto focuses on consuming exactly what you need. If you use a great Keto plan, your body will lack no nutrients and will not suffer any deficiency.

Reduced hunger

The reason we find it hard to stick to diets is hunger. It doesn't matter your age; diets do not become easier to stick to. We may have a mental picture of the healthy body we want. We may even have clear visuals of the kind of life we want to leave once free from unhealthy living but none of that matters when hunger enters the scene. However, Keto diet is a diet that combats this problem. Keto diet focuses on consuming plenty of proteins. Proteins are filling and do not let you feel hungry too easily. In addition, when your carb levels are reduced, your appetite takes a hit. It is a win-win situation.

Weight loss

Keto not only burns fat, but it also reduces that crave for food. Combined, these are two great ways to lose weight. It is one of the diets that has proven to help the most when it comes to weight loss. The Keto diet has been proven to be one of the best ways to burn stubborn belly fat while keeping yourself revitalized and healthy.

Reduces blood sugar and insulin

After 50, monitoring blood sugar can be a real struggle. Cutting down on cars drastically reduces both insulin levels and blood sugar levels. This means that the Keto diet will benefit millions as a lot of people struggle with insulin complications and high blood sugar levels. It has been proven to help as when some people embark on Keto, they cut up to half of the carbs they consume. It's a treasure for those with diabetes and insulin resistance. A study was carried out on people with type 2 diabetes. After cutting down on carbs, within six months, 95 percent of the people were able to reduce or totally stop using their glucose-lowering medication

Lower levels of triglycerides

A lot of people do not know what triglycerides are. Triglycerides are molecules of fat in your blood. They are known to circulate the bloodstream and can be very dangerous. High levels of triglycerides can cause heart failures and heart diseases. However, Keto is known to reduce these levels.

Reduces acne

Although acne is mostly suffered by those who are young, there are cases of people above 50 having it. Moreover, Keto is not only for persons after 50. Acne is not only caused by blocked pores. There are quite a number of things proven to cause it. One of these things is your blood sugar. When you consume processed and refined carbs, it affects gut bacteria and results in the fluctuation of blood sugar levels. When the gut bacteria and sugar levels are affected, the skin suffers. However, when you embark on the Keto diet, you cut off on carbs intake which means that in the very first place, your gut bacteria will not be affected thereby cutting off that avenue to develop.

Increases hdl levels

HDL refers to high-density lipoprotein. When your HDL levels are compared to your LDL levels and are not found low, your risk of developing a heart disease is lowered. This is great for persons over 50 as heart diseases suddenly become more probable. Eating fats and reducing your intake of carbohydrates is one of the most assured ways to increase your high-density lipoprotein levels.

Reduces ldl levels

High levels of LDL can be very problematic when you attain 50. This is because LDL refers to bad cholesterol. People with high levels of this cholesterol are more likely to get heart attacks. When you reduce the number of carbs you consume, you will increase the size of bad LDL particles. However, this will result in the reduction of the total LDL particles as they would have increased in size. Smaller LDL particles have been linked to heart diseases while larger ones have been proven to have lower risks attached.

May help combat cancer

I termed this under 'may' because research on this is not as extensive and conclusive as we would like it to be. However, there is proof supporting it. Firstly, it helps reduce the levels of blood sugar which in turn reduces insulin complications which in turn reduces the risk of developing cancers related to insulin levels. In addition, Keto places more oxidative stress on cancer cells than on normal cells thereby making it great for chemotherapy. The risk of developing cancer after fifty is still existent and so, Keto is literally a lifesaver.

May lower blood pressure

High blood pressure plagues adults much more than it does young ones. Once you attain 50, you must monitor your blood pressure rates. Reduction in the intake of carbohydrates is a proven way to lower your blood pressure. When you cut down on your carbs and lower your blood sugar levels, you greatly reduce your chances of getting some other diseases.

Combats metabolic syndrome

As you grow older, you may find that you struggle to control your blood sugar level. Metabolic syndrome is another condition that has been proven to have an influence on diabetes and heart disease development. The symptoms associated with metabolic syndrome include but are not limited to high triglycerides, obesity, high blood sugar level, and low levels of high-density lipoprotein cholesterol.

However, you will find that reducing your level of carbohydrate intake greatly affects this. You will improve your health and majorly attack all the above-listed symptoms. Keto diet helps to fight against metabolic syndrome which is a big win.

Great for the heart

People over the age of 50 have been proven to have more chances of developing heart diseases. Keto diet has been proven to be great for the heart. As it increases good cholesterol levels and reduces the levels of bad cholesterol, you will find that partaking in the Keto diet proves extremely beneficial for your health.

May reduce seizure risks

When you change your intake levels the combination of protein, fat, and carbs, as we explained before, your body will go into ketosis. Ketosis has been proven to reduce seizure levels in people who suffer from epilepsy. When they do not respond to treatment, the ketosis treatment is used. This has been done for decades.

Combats brain disorders

Keto doesn't end there, it also combats Alzheimer's and Parkinson's disease. There are some parts of your brain that can only burn glucose and so, your body needs it. If you do not consume carbs, your lover will make use of protein to produce glucose. Your brain can also burn ketones. Ketones are formed when your carb level is very low. With this, the ketogenic diet has been used f r plenty of years to treat epilepsy in children who aren't responding to drugs. For adults, it can work the same magic as it is now being linked to treating Alzheimer's and Parkinson's disease

Helps women suffering from polycystic ovarian syndrome

This syndrome affects women of all ages. PCOS is short for polycystic ovarian syndrome. Polycystic ovarian syndrome is an endocrine disorder that results in enlarged ovaries with cysts. These cysts are dangerous and cause other complications. It has been proven that a high intake of carbohydrates negatively affects women suffering from polycystic ovarian syndrome. When a woman with PCOS cuts down on carbs and embarks on the Keto diet, the polycystic ovarian syndrome falls under attack.

It is beyond doubt that the Keto diet is beneficial in so many ways that it almost looks unreal. If you are to embark on the Keto diet, there are several things you must know.

Caution for Keto

Yes, Keto is beneficial and yes, it has a lot of benefits, but it is no small thing and so, it must be approached with caution. Here are some tips you should keep in mind before embarking on Keto.

Make use of recipes you can trust

Keto involves a lot of meal planning and this single phase is where a lot of people get it wrong. Your meals are no longer allowed to be careless and you must note everything that goes into your mouth. If you are embarking on a Keto diet, you must use recipes you can trust. The recipes must be beneficial, safe, and delicious. Keto should not take out the enjoyment in your meals.

You may need a doctor

If you have had any issue with blood sugar, insulin levels or diabetes, consult your doctor before embarking on Keto. Do not make any dietary changes as large as Keto to your diet without first informing your doctor. He or she is in the best position to guide you properly. See your doctor.

It will be hard at first

Keto is no walk in the park. However, people continue on the path of Keto despite the initial difficulty because the results are evident after a short while. When you kick-start Keto, you may suffer from low blood sugar, sluggishness, and constipation, However, they will all wear off in a few days if you are religious about it.

Can Keto have side effects?

Yes. Keto can have side effects. Keto can have negative side effects if it is wrongly done. Keto cuts down on carbs and replaces them with fat. However, if the replacement is not adequately carried out, a lot of negative side effects may occur.

If you do not make use of quality meal plans and recipes, you'll lack nutrients that your body needs. With Keto, you must not lack proteins and so, your meals must be planned.

How to reach ketosis

Reaching the state of ketosis is not so straightforward for many people. In order to effectively reach ketosis, there are some steps you must take.

Eat the right food- Ketosis relies a lot on what you eat. To reach ketosis, you need to first cut down on the carbohydrates you take in. Secondly, you need to take in much more fats in your diets. However, you should just take in any fat, you should make sure to take in healthy fat. Taking in unhealthy fats can cause more harm than good.

Exercise- To efficiently reach ketosis, you should make sure to exercise. It doesn't have to be intensive, however, long walks, jugs, biking, and other exercises can help your body reach ketosis.

Try intermittent fasting- Some people combine intermittent fasting with ketosis. The reason is that, as you progress, your hunger pangs are reduced greatly, and you will find intermittent fasting easy. In fact, even when you do not plan to, you'll find yourself doing it. It is definitely not compulsory but if you are making use of ketosis to lose weight, intermittent fasting is a great bonus.

Take lots of fruits and vegetables- Fruits and vegetables for snacks will keep your body healthy and help revitalize your skin.

Include coconut oil in your diet- Coconut is compulsory if you want to reach ketosis. Coconut oil contains healthy fat. It helps the body reach ketosis and contains four types of MCTs. It is one of the best tools for inducing ketosis. If you have never made use of coconut oil before, start slowly and increase your intake gradually.

CHAPTER 7:

The Tips And Tricks That Help You Contain Diabetes.

Tips for Reversing Diabetes

Exercise for diabetics

The most recommended type of exercise for diabetics is aerobic conditioning exercise. This kind of exercise keeps the heart rate up and sustains that heart rate level for 20 to 30 minutes. The types of exercise recommended for this include treadmill sessions, brisk walking, jogging, swimming and cycling. Start slow and when you reach a level wherein you feel your heart rate is pumped up, maintain the pace for at least 20 to 30 minutes. This should have at least 5 to 10 minutes of warm-up and cool-down.

Experts recommend performing the exercise at least 4 to 6 times a week. Rest days should be placed in between exercise days, but not in two consecutive days. It would be ideal to work on an exercise program with a trainer in order to properly assess and monitor progress, heart rate levels and period of exercise.

Diet plans for diabetics

According to nutritionist Diane Lara of the Whitaker Wellness Institute, the key to a proper diabetic diet is low sweet and low sodium levels on food. So, the first thing that a diabetic need to do is to remove all the refined sweeteners in the kitchen and drastically reduce salt in food. Sounds mortifying? Relax. Of course, food wouldn't be as appetizing without these taste enhancers that's why there are acceptable substitutes.

Suggested alternative sweeteners:

Stevia - a plant-derived sweetener extracted from the plant Stevia rebaudiana. It is a hundred times sweeter than regular sugar that's why a pinch of it would usually be enough to sweeten a cup of coffee. It has zero calories and does not elevate blood sugar levels.

Xylitol – a chemical sweetener obtained from birch trees, but also found naturally from the fibers of various types of vegetables, fruits, berries and mushrooms. It has 40 percent fewer calories than regular table sugar and is absorbed slowly by the body.

Brown rice syrup – As the name suggests, this natural sweetener is derived from brown rice. The body slowly metabolizes it and therefore does not cause a spike in blood sugar levels.

Salt Substitutes:

Vegetable seasoning – This seasoning comes from dehydrated grains, vegetables and fruits, but without the salt. The mixture will contain natural sodium so it will still taste a little salty because of the mixture of the ingredients. However, it won't be as salty as the regular table salt. Therefore, the trick is to use twice or thrice more of the seasoning to reach the desired saltiness or flavor.

NuSalt or NoSalt (Potassium chloride) –This product that is available in most grocery stores contains potassium chloride and zero sodium. Potassium helps balance sodium levels in the body, protecting it from heart disease, high blood pressure and stroke.

Tips Maintaining Your Progress

Fighting diabetes is a lifetime commitment. Even if your blood glucose levels have normalized, it does not mean that you can go back to an idle lifestyle and eat the wrong foods. Slacking will surely bring back the symptoms. However, if you commit to doing aerobic exercises and a diabetes-friendly eating program for at least 30 days, it will jumpstart your path towards healthy living for the rest of your life.

Remember it only takes 30 days to commit to this and you can change your health forever. Just commit to two things for the following 30 days: 30 minutes of exercise every day and eating only your choice of diabetic-friendly meals for 30 days.

You should also check your progress regularly to ensure you are doing things right. Eating healthy foods and exercising for the following 30 days will surely make you look and feel a lot better. However, if you are a diabetic, you cannot base the evidence that your health is getting better merely on whether you gained weight, lost weight or look healthier. Blood sugar levels constantly need to be checked.

Use a Glucose Monitoring Device

This is a small handy digital unit that you can easily buy in a pharmacy. A sterile needle (lancet) is used to prick the tip of a finger to draw a drop of blood to be placed in the test strip. The strip is then inserted in the digital device and will read the blood glucose level within just a few seconds. Blood is drawn out of the fingertips because it is the area in the body that reacts fastest to changes in glucose levels.

There are also different types of glucose monitoring devices that can test the forearms, thighs, the base of the thumb and the upper arm. For diabetics, blood glucose levels should ideally be checked several times throughout the day. Some check it every time they feel symptoms kicking in such as cravings, frequent urinations or extreme sleepiness after consuming a meal.

Get in touch with your doctor for regular check-ups

The type of doctor you should be seeing if you happen to have diabetes is an Endocrinologist because they have a special training in treating people with diabetes. However, to ensure complete overall care, there should be a team of doctors and experts you should be visiting regularly who can help you manage various symptoms. These include a primary care doctor, a dietician, an eye doctor, a dentist, a podiatrist, a physical trainer, and a diabetes educator.

CHAPTER 8:

Shopping List

Here's the best part about the list there are no strange or rare fruits in it just your normal everyday fruits you see around you that are tasty but also contain the nutrient needed to manage blood glucose, lose weight and control your cholesterol level from building up to dangerous condition.

Here is why this is important you can eat these foods for breakfast lunch and dinner by combining it in different ratio or parts.

SOURCE FOR VEGETABLES FOODS

Tomatoes

Broccoli

Spinach

Pumpkin

Ginger

Garlic

caution the use of Garlic and ginger should be limited if you're at risk of high blood pressure, also pregnant women and breast-feeding mothers and also if you're on medication you should avoid using them without doctors' consent because of their antioxidant and medicinal nature.

Bell Peppers

Hot Peppers

Cauliflower

Leeks

Asparagus

Cabbage

Swiss Chard

Kale

Winter Squash

Carrots

Beets

SOURCE OF PROTEIN/STARCH FOODS

Eggs

Avocado

Beans

Lentils

Spirulina

Nuts/Seeds Foods

Pistachios

Almonds

Walnuts

Chia Seed

Flax Seed

OTHER FOODS

Dark Chocolate however, there's a Caveat and here's the trickiest part dark chocolate has different varieties some are packed with sugars, fructose and artificial

Sweeteners, therefore, ensure you eat chocolate with brands that contain more cacao, Maca and less Ingredients that ends with –ose. Syrups corns etc.

Other includes:

Mushrooms

Olive Oil

FRUITS FOODS

Blueberries

Strawberries

Cranberries

Pomegranates

Cherries

Bananas

Cantaloupe

Pineapple has a little precaution, avoid eating overripe pineapple because it's easily converted to glucose in the blood stream, which leads to increase in insulin in the blood. Therefore, pineapple apart from its great source of vitamin should be limited because it contains less Fiber compare to its sugar content so also with watermelon.

Apples

Kiwi

Apricots

Grapes

Lemon

Lime

Oranges

Papaya

Mango

Peaches

GRAINS FOODS

Quinoa

Brown Rice

Rolled Oats

Kefir

Wheat Germ

DAIRY FOODS

Greek Yogurt

DRINKS FOODS

Green Tea

Water

Fish salmon and Sandrine's

Salmon: should be sea salmon and not reared from anywhere else. Therefore, if you can avoid eating reared salmon, please avoid.

LIST YOU SHOULD NEVER EAT

Like a hamster on a wheel you need to avoid these foods like the plague and also tell you families and friends in the most loving ways you can. Here's why because most times our families and friends want the best for us however, in their bid to show love and empathies with us they could buy foods that will not only harm, but also prove to have lifelong effect to your overall health, and increase your risks to chronic conditions and degenerative diseases.

Therefore, you need to make it known to others about the treats and gift you'll accept and those you don't of course in a loving and kind way. My friend's daughter calls it a gingerly way.

Enough of these talks here's the gist that could aggravate your condition that you will frequently eat or offered by families and friends.

This list contains food that you might at first glance think they should be great for you, however, their sugar content and the glycemic index makes them unsuitable for your condition as a diabetic because they are easily to digest, and have high glycemic index therefore, you've to avoid consuming them no matter how hard it might seem at first, or limit the amount you consume and find other great alternatives.

That said here's the list although this is not the list under the sun because new research and studies are on the way.

With all that said, here's a list of foods to avoid because of their glycemic index, ease of digestion, and health benefits.

Sodas in whatever brand, shape or form should be avoided because of their high sugar content that's easy to get into the blood stream,

processed food and fries

products containing Fructose

Corn Syrups in whatever brand.

Sugars and product containing artificial flavors.

I know it's very hard to avoid these foods without the cravings or trying to motivate yourself to eat, that's why I've shared an elaborate method how to avoid, minimize or cut sugar cravings forever.

CHAPTER 9:

Breakfast

Granola with Fruits

Preparation Time: 15 minutes

Cooking Time: 35 minutes

Servings: 6

Ingredients:

3 cups quick cooking oats

1 cup almonds, sliced

½ cup wheat germ

3 tablespoons butter

1 teaspoon ground cinnamon

1 cup honey

3 cups whole grain cereal flakes

½ cup raisins

½ cup dried cranberries

½ cup dates, pitted and chopped

Directions:

Preheat your oven to 325 degrees F.

Arrange the almonds and oats on a baking sheet.

Bake for 15 minutes.

Mix the wheat germ, butter, cinnamon and honey in a bowl.

Add the toasted almonds and oats.

Mix well.

Spread on the baking sheet.

Bake for 20 minutes.

Mix with the rest of the ingredients.

Let cool and serve.

Nutrition:

Calories 210

Total Fat 7 g

Saturated Fat 2 g

Cholesterol 5 mg

Sodium 58 mg

Total Carbohydrate 36 g

Dietary Fiber 4 g

Total Sugars 2 g

Protein 5 g

Potassium 250 mg

Apple & Cinnamon Pancake

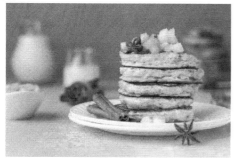

Preparation Time: 15 minutes

Cooking Time: 10 minutes

Servings: 4

Ingredients:

¼ teaspoon ground cinnamon

1 ¾ cups Better Baking Mix

1 tablespoon oil

1 cup water

2 egg whites

½ cup sugar-free applesauce

Cooking spray

1 cup plain yogurt

Sugar substitute

Directions:

Blend the cinnamon and the baking mix in a bowl.

Create a hole in the middle and add the oil, water, egg and applesauce.

Mix well.

Spray your pan with oil.

Place it on medium heat.

Pour ¼ cup of the batter.

Flip the pancake and cook until golden.

Serve with yogurt and sugar substitute.

Nutrition:

Calories 231

Total Fat 6 g

Saturated Fat 1 g

Cholesterol 54 mg

Sodium 545 mg

Total Carbohydrate 37 g

Dietary Fiber 4 g

Total Sugars 1 g

Protein 8 g

Potassium 750 mg

Spinach Scramble

Preparation Time: 5 minutes

Cooking Time: 15 minutes

Servings: 2

Ingredients:

¼ cup liquid egg substitute

¼ cup skim milk

Salt and pepper to taste

2 tablespoons crumbled bacon

13 ½ oz. canned spinach, drained

Cooking spray

Directions:

Mix all the ingredients in a large bowl.

Pour the mixture on a pan greased with oil, placed over medium heat.

Stir until fully cooked.

Calories: 70 calories, Carbohydrates: 5 g, Protein: 8 g, Fat: 2 g, Saturated Fat: 1 g, Sodium: 700 mg, Fiber: 2 g

Nutrition:

Calories 70

Total Fat 2 g

Saturated Fat 1 g

Cholesterol 25 mg

Sodium 700 mg

Total Carbohydrate 5 g

Dietary Fiber 2 g

Total Sugars 1 g

Protein 8 g - Potassium 564 mg

Breakfast Parfait

Preparation Time: 5 minutes

Cooking Time: 0 minute

Servings: 2

Ingredients:

4 oz. unsweetened applesauce

6 oz. non-fat and sugar-free vanilla yogurt

¼ teaspoon pumpkin pie spice

¼ teaspoon honey

1 cup low-fat granola

Directions:

Mix all the ingredients except the granola in a bowl. Layer the mixture with the granola in a cup. Refrigerate before serving.

Nutrition:

Calories 287 - Total Fat 3 g

Saturated Fat 1 g - Cholesterol 28 mg

Sodium 186 mg

Total Carbohydrate 57 g

Dietary Fiber 4 g - Total Sugars 2 g

Protein 8 g - Potassium 450 mg

Asparagus & Cheese Omelet

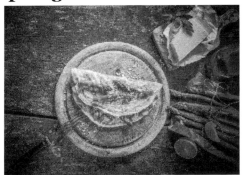

Preparation Time: 10 minutes

Cooking Time: 10 minutes

Servings: 2

Ingredients:

Cooking spray

4 spears asparagus, sliced

Pepper to taste

3 egg whites

½ teaspoon olive oil

1 oz. spreadable cheese, sliced

1 teaspoon parsley, chopped

Directions:

Spray oil on your pan.

Cook asparagus on the pan over medium high heat for 5 to 7 minutes.

Wrap with foil and set aside.

In a bowl, mix pepper and egg whites.

Add olive oil to the pan.

Add the egg whites.

When you start to see the sides forming, add the asparagus and cheese on top.

Use a spatula to lift and fold the egg.

Sprinkle parsley on top before serving.

Nutrition:

Calories 119

Total Fat 5 g

Saturated Fat 2 g

Cholesterol 10 mg

Sodium 427 mg

Total Carbohydrate 5 g

Dietary Fiber 2 g

Total Sugars 3 g

Protein 15 g

Potassium 308 mg

Sausage, Egg & Potatoes

Preparation Time: 15 minutes

Cooking Time: 10 hours and 10 minutes

Servings: 6

Ingredients:

Cooking spray

12 oz. chicken sausage links, sliced

1 onion, sliced into wedges

2 red sweet peppers, sliced into strips

1 ½ lb. potatoes, sliced into strips

¼ cup low-sodium chicken broth

Black pepper to taste

½ teaspoon dried thyme, crushed

6 eggs

½ cup low-fat cheddar cheese, shredded

Directions:

Spray oil on a heavy foil sheet.

Put the sausage, onion, sweet peppers and potatoes on the foil.

Drizzle top with the chicken broth.

Season with the pepper and thyme.

Fold to seal.

Place the packet inside a cooker.

Cook on low setting for 10 hours.

Meanwhile, boil the egg until fully cooked.

Serve eggs with the sausage mixture.

Nutrition:

Calories 281

Total Fat 12 g

Saturated Fat 4 g

Cholesterol 262 mg

Sodium 485 mg

Total Carbohydrate 23 g

Dietary Fiber 3 g

Total Sugars 3 g

Protein 21 g

Potassium 262 mg

Cucumber & Yogurt

Preparation Time: 5 minutes

Cooking Time: 0 minute

Servings: 1

Ingredients:

1 cup low-fat yogurt

½ cup cucumber, diced

¼ teaspoon lemon zest

¼ teaspoon lemon juice

¼ teaspoon fresh mint, chopped

Salt to taste

Directions:

Mix all the ingredients in a jar.

Refrigerate and serve.

Nutrition:

Calories 164

Total Fat 4 g

Saturated Fat 2 g

Cholesterol 15 mg

Sodium 318 mg

Total Carbohydrate 19 g

Dietary Fiber 1 g

Total Sugars 18 g

Protein 13 g

Potassium 683 mg

Yogurt Breakfast Pudding

Preparation Time: 8 hours and 10 minutes

Cooking Time: 0 minute

Servings: 2

Ingredients:

½ cup rolled oats

6 oz. low-fat yogurt

¼ cup canned pineapple

½ cup fat-free milk

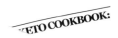

½ teaspoon vanilla

⅛ teaspoon ground cinnamon

1 tablespoon flaxseed meal

4 teaspoons almonds, toasted and sliced

½ cup apple, chopped

Directions:

In a bowl, mix all the ingredients except almonds and apple.

Transfer the mixture into an airtight container.

Cover with the lid and refrigerate for 8 hours.

Top with the almonds and apple before serving.

Nutrition:

Calories 255

Total Fat 7 g

Saturated Fat 1 g

Cholesterol 5 mg

Sodium 84 mg

Total Carbohydrate 38 g

Dietary Fiber 5 g

Total Sugars 21 g

Protein 11 g

Potassium 345 mg

Vegetable Omelet

Preparation Time: 5 minutes

Cooking Time: 25 minutes

Servings: 4

Ingredients:

½ cup yellow summer squash, chopped

½ cup canned diced tomatoes with herbs, drained

½ ripe avocado, pitted and chopped

½ cup cucumber, chopped

2 eggs

2 tablespoons water

Salt and pepper to taste

1 teaspoon dried basil, crushed

Cooking spray

¼ cup low-fat Monterey Jack cheese, shredded

Chives, chopped

Directions:

In a bowl, mix the squash, tomatoes, avocado and cucumber.

In another bowl, mix the eggs, water, salt, pepper and basil.

Spray oil on a pan over medium heat.

Pour egg mixture on the pan.

Put the vegetable mixture on top of the egg.

Lift and fold.

until the egg has set.

Sprinkle cheese and chives on top.

Nutrition:

Calories 128

Total Fat 6 g

Saturated Fat 2 g

Cholesterol 97 mg

Sodium 357 mg

Total Carbohydrate 7 g

Dietary Fiber 3 g

Total Sugars 4 g

Protein 12 g

Potassium 341 mg

Almond & Berry Smoothie

Preparation Time: 10 minutes

Cooking Time: 0 minute

Serving: 1

Ingredients:

⅔ cup frozen raspberries

½ cup frozen banana, sliced

½ cup almond milk (unsweetened)

3 tablespoons almonds, sliced

¼ teaspoon ground cinnamon

⅛ teaspoon vanilla extract

¼ cup blueberries

1 tablespoon coconut flakes (unsweetened)

Directions:

Put all the ingredients in a blender except coconut flakes. Pulse until smooth.

Top with the coconut flakes before serving.

Nutrition:

Calories 360

Total Fat 19 g

Saturated Fat 3 g

Cholesterol 0 mg

Sodium 89 mg

Total Carbohydrate 46 g

Dietary Fiber 14 g

Total Sugars 21 g

Protein 9 g

Potassium 736 mg

Easy Veggie Muffins

Preparation time: 10 minutes

Cooking time: 40 minutes

Servings: 4

Ingredients:

¾ cup cheddar cheese, shredded

1 cup green onion, chopped

1 cup tomatoes, chopped

1 cup broccoli, chopped

2 cups non-fat milk

1 cup biscuit ix

4 eggs

Cooking spray

1 teaspoon Italian seasoning

A pinch of black pepper

Directions:

Grease a muffin tray with cooking spray and divide broccoli, tomatoes cheese and onions in each muffin cup.

In a bowl, combine green onions with milk, biscuit mix, eggs, pepper and Italian seasoning, whisk well and pour towards the muffin tray also.

Cook the muffins within the oven at 375 degrees F for 40 minutes, divide them between plates and serve.

Enjoy!

Nutrition:

calories 216

fat 6

fiber 6

carbs 16

protein 6

Carrot Muffins

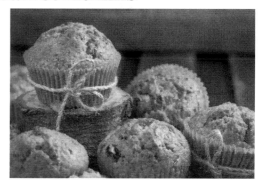

Preparation time: 10 minutes

Cooking Time: 30 minutes

Servings: 5

Ingredients:

1 and ½ cups whole-wheat flour

½ cup stevia

1 teaspoon baking powder

½ teaspoon cinnamon powder

½ teaspoon baking soda

¼ cup natural apple juice

¼ cup organic essential olive oil

1 egg

1 cup fresh cranberries

2 carrots, grated

2 teaspoons ginger, grated

¼ cup pecans, chopped

Cooking spray

Directions:

In a substantial bowl, combine the flour because of the stevia, baking powder, cinnamon and baking soda and stir well.

Add apple juice, oil, egg, cranberries, carrots, ginger and pecans and stir rather well.

Grease a muffin tray with cooking spray, divide the muffin mix, introduce inside oven and cook at 375 degrees F for half an hour.

Divide the muffins between plates and serve enjoying.

Enjoy!

Nutrition:

calories 216

fat 6

fiber 6

carbs 16

protein 6

Pineapple Oatmeal

Preparation time: 10 minutes

Cooking time: 25 minutes

Servings: 4

Ingredients:

2 cups old-fashioned oats

1 cup walnuts, chopped

2 cups pineapple, cubed

1 tablespoon ginger, grated

2 cups non-fat milk

2 eggs

2 tablespoons stevia

2 teaspoons vanilla flavor

Directions:

In a bowl, combine the oats while using the pineapple, walnuts and ginger, stir and divide into 4 ramekins.

In a bowl, combine the milk using the eggs, stevia and vanilla, whisk well and pour about the oats mix.

Introduce inside oven and cook at 400 degrees F for 25 minutes. Serve enjoying. Enjoy!

Nutrition:

calories 216

fat 6

fiber 6

carbs 16

protein 6

Spinach Muffins

Preparation time: 10 minutes

Cooking time: 30 minutes

Servings: 6

Ingredients:

6 eggs

½ cup non-fat milk

1 cup low-fat cheese, crumbled

4 ounces spinach

½ cup roasted red pepper, chopped

2 ounces prosciutto, chopped

Cooking spray

Directions:

In a bowl, combine the eggs using the milk, cheese, spinach, red pepper and prosciutto and whisk well.

Grease a muffin tray with cooking spray, divide the muffin mix, introduce within the oven and bake at 350 degrees F for around 30 minutes.

Divide between plates and serve enjoying.

Enjoy!

Nutrition:

calories 156

fat 16

fiber 6

carbs 6

protein 10

Chia Seeds Breakfast Mix

Preparation time: 8 hours

Cooking time: 0 minutes

Servings: 4

Ingredients:

2 cups old-fashioned oats

4 tablespoons chia seeds

4 tablespoons coconut sugar

3 cups coconut milk

1 teaspoon lemon zest, grated

1 cup blueberries

Directions:

In a bowl, combine the oats with chia seeds, sugar, milk, lemon zest and blueberries, stir, and divide into cups whilst within the fridge for 8 hours.

Serve enjoying.

Enjoy!

Nutrition:

calories 286

fat 16

fiber 6

carbs 16

protein 8

Breakfast Fruits Bowls

Preparation time: 10 minutes

Cooking time: 0 minutes

Servings: 2

Ingredients:

1 cup mango, chopped

1 banana, sliced

1 cup pineapple, chopped

1 cup almond milk

Directions:

In a bowl, combine the mango with all the current banana, pineapple and almond milk, stir, divide into smaller bowls and serve each day.

Enjoy!

Nutrition:

calories 186

fat 6

fiber 6

carbs 16

protein 6

Pumpkin Breakfast Cookies

Preparation time: 10 minutes

Cooking time: 25 minutes

Servings: 6

Ingredients:

2 cups whole-wheat grains flour

1 cup old-fashioned oats

1 teaspoon baking soda

1 teaspoon pumpkin pie spice

15 ounces pumpkin puree

1 cup coconut oil, melted

1 cup coconut sugar

1 egg

½ cup pepitas, roasted

½ cup cherries, dried

Directions:

In a bowl, combine the flour with the oats, baking soda, pumpkin spice, pumpkin puree, oil, sugar, egg, pepitas and cherries, stir well, shape medium cookies for this reason mix, stick them all about the lined baking sheet, introduce inside oven and bake at 350 degrees F for 25 minutes.

Serve the cookies enjoying.

Enjoy!

Nutrition:

calories 286

fat 16

fiber 6 - carbs 16

protein 6

Veggie Scramble

Preparation time: 10 minutes

Cooking time: 2 minutes

Servings: 1

Ingredients:

1 egg

1 tablespoon water

¼ cup broccoli, chopped

¼ cup mushrooms, chopped

A pinch of black pepper

1 tablespoon low-fat mozzarella, shredded

1 tablespoon walnuts, chopped

Cooking spray

Directions:

Grease a ramekin with cooking spray, add the egg, water, pepper, mushrooms and broccoli and whisk well.

Introduce inside microwave and cook for two main minutes.

Add mozzarella and walnuts on top and serve every day.

Enjoy!

Nutrition:

calories 216

fat 6

fiber 6

carbs 16

protein 6

Quinoa Bowls

Preparation time: 10 minutes

Cooking time: 5 minutes

Servings: 4

Ingredients:

1 and ½ cups water

1 teaspoon cinnamon powder

1 and ½ cups quinoa

¼ cup raisins

¾ cup apple, cored, peeled and chopped

1 cup apple juice

1 cup non-fat yogurt

¼ cup pistachios, chopped

Directions:

In your instant pot, combine the water with the cinnamon, quinoa, raisins, apple, apple juice, yogurt and pistachios, stir, cover and cook on High for 5 minutes.

Stir the quinoa mix one more time, divide into bowls and serve for breakfast.

Enjoy!

Nutrition:

calories 196

fat 6

fiber 6

carbs 16

protein 6

Delicious Yogurt and Fruits

Preparation time: 10 minutes

Cooking time: 10 minutes

Servings: 4

Ingredients:

4 cups non-fat yogurt

1 tablespoon vanilla bean paste

½ cup pears, chopped

½ cup cherries, pitted and halved

4 tablespoons coconut sugar

Directions:

In your instant pot, mix the yogurt with the vanilla bean paste, pears, cherries and coconut sugar, stir, cover, cook on Low for 10 minutes, divide into bowls and serve for breakfast.

Enjoy!

Nutrition:

calories 156

fat 6

fiber 6

carbs 16

protein 5

Easy Breakfast Fruit Mix

Preparation time: 10 minutes

Cooking time: 10 minutes

Servings: 4

Ingredients:

1 pear, chopped

1 plum, pitted and chopped

1 apple, cored and chopped

3 tablespoons coconut oil, melted

½ teaspoon cinnamon powder

¼ cup unsweetened coconut, shredded

2 tablespoons sunflower seeds, toasted

Directions:

Add the oil to your instant pot, add pear, plum, apple, cinnamon, coconut and sunflower seeds, toss, cover, cook on High for 10 minutes, divide into bowls and serve.

Enjoy!

Nutrition:

calories 176

fat 6

fiber 6

carbs 16

protein 6

Breakfast Apples Mix

Preparation time: 10 minutes

Cooking time: 8 minutes

Servings: 6

Ingredients:

6 apples, cored and cut into wedges

1 cup natural apple juice

½ cup coconut sugar

2 tablespoons cinnamon powder

Directions:

In your instant pot, mix the apples with apple juice, sugar and cinnamon, toss, cover and cook on High for 8 minutes.

Divide into bowls and serve for breakfast.

Enjoy!

Nutrition:

calories 176

fat 6

fiber 6

carbs 16

protein 6

Veggie Quiche

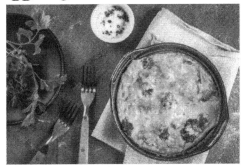

Preparation time: 6 minutes

Cooking time: 55 minutes

Servings: 8

Ingredients:

½ cup sun-dried tomatoes, chopped

1 prepared pie crust

2 tablespoons avocado oil

1 yellow onion, chopped

2 garlic cloves, minced

2 cups spinach, chopped

1 red bell pepper, chopped

¼ cup kalamata olives, pitted and sliced

1 teaspoon parsley flakes

1 teaspoon oregano, dried

1/3 cup feta cheese, crumbled

4 eggs, whisked

1 and ½ cups almond milk

1 cup cheddar cheese, shredded

Salt and black pepper to the taste

Directions:

Heat up a pan with the oil over medium-high heat, add the garlic and onion and sauté for 3 minutes.

Add the bell pepper and sauté for 3 minutes more.

Add the olives, parsley, spinach, oregano, salt and pepper and cook everything for 5 minutes.

Add tomatoes and the cheese, toss and take off the heat.

Arrange the pie crust in a pie plate, pour the spinach and tomatoes mix inside and spread.

In a bowl, mix the eggs with salt, pepper, the milk and half of the cheese, whisk and pour over the mixture in the pie crust.

Sprinkle the remaining cheese on top and bake at 375 degrees F for 40 minutes.

Cool the quiche down, slice and serve for breakfast.

Nutrition:

calories 216

fat 16

fiber 6

carbs 16

protein 6

Potato Hash

Preparation time: 10 minutes

Cooking time: 15 minutes

Servings: 4

Ingredients:

A drizzle of olive oil

2 gold potatoes, cubed

2 garlic cloves, minced

1 yellow onion, chopped

1 cup canned chickpeas, drained

Salt and black pepper to the taste

1 and ½ teaspoon allspice, ground

1-pound baby asparagus, trimmed and chopped

1 teaspoon sweet paprika

1 teaspoon oregano, dried

1 teaspoon coriander, ground

2 tomatoes, cubed

1 cup parsley, chopped

½ cup feta cheese, crumbled

Directions:

Heat up a pan with a drizzle of oil over medium-high heat, add the potatoes, onion, garlic, salt and pepper and cook for 7 minutes.

Add the rest of the ingredients except the tomatoes, parsley and the cheese, toss, cook for 7 more minutes and transfer to a bowl.

Add the remaining ingredients, toss and serve for breakfast.

Nutrition:

calories 536

fat 26

fiber 6

carbs 36

protein 26

Leeks and Eggs Muffins

Preparation time: 10 minutes

Cooking time: 20 minutes

Servings: 2

Ingredients:

3 eggs, whisked

¼ cup baby spinach

2 tablespoons leeks, chopped

4 tablespoons parmesan, grated

2 tablespoons almond milk

Cooking spray

1 small red bell pepper, chopped

Salt and black pepper to the taste

1 tomato, cubed

2 tablespoons cheddar cheese, grated

Directions:

In a bowl, combine the eggs with the milk, salt, pepper and the rest of the ingredients except the cooking spray and whisk well.

Grease a muffin tin with the cooking spray and divide the eggs mixture in each muffin mould.

Bake at 380 degrees F for 20 minutes and serve them for breakfast.

Nutrition:

calories 306

fat 16

fiber 6

carbs 6

protein 24

CHAPTER 10:

Lunch Recipes

Pork Chops with Grape Sauce

Preparation Time: 15 minutes

Cooking Time: 25 minutes

Servings: 4

Ingredients:

Cooking spray

4 pork chops

¼ cup onion, sliced

1 clove garlic, minced

½ cup low-sodium chicken broth

¾ cup apple juice

1 tablespoon cornstarch

1 tablespoon balsamic vinegar

1 teaspoon honey

1 cup seedless red grapes, sliced in half

Directions:

Spray oil on your pan.

Put it over medium heat.

Add the pork chops to the pan.

Cook for 5 minutes per side.

Remove and set aside.

Add onion and garlic.

Cook for 2 minutes.

Pour in the broth and apple juice.

Bring to a boil.

Reduce heat to simmer.

Put the pork chops back to the skillet.

Simmer for 4 minutes.

In a bowl, mix the cornstarch, vinegar and honey.

Add to the pan.

Cook until the sauce has thickened.

Add the grapes.

Pour sauce over the pork chops before serving.

Nutrition:

Calories 188

Total Fat 4 g

Saturated Fat 1 g

Cholesterol 47 mg

Sodium 117 mg

Total Carbohydrate 18 g

Dietary Fiber 1 g

Total Sugars 13 g

Protein 19 g

Potassium 759 mg

Roasted Pork & Apples

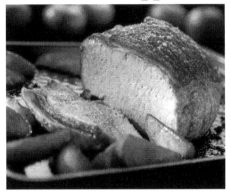

Preparation Time: 15 minutes

Cooking Time: 30 minutes

Servings: 4

Ingredients:

Salt and pepper to taste

½ teaspoon dried, crushed

1 lb. pork tenderloin

1 tablespoon canola oil

1 onion, sliced into wedges

3 cooking apples, sliced into wedges

⅔ cup apple cider

Sprigs fresh sage

Directions:

In a bowl, mix salt, pepper and sage.

Season both sides of pork with this mixture.

Place a pan over medium heat.

Brown both sides.

Transfer to a roasting pan.

Add the onion on top and around the pork.

Drizzle oil on top of the pork and apples.

Roast in the oven at 425 degrees F for 10 minutes.

Add the apples, roast for another 15 minutes.

In a pan, boil the apple cider and then simmer for 10 minutes.

Pour the apple cider sauce over the pork before serving.

Nutrition:

Calories 239

Total Fat 6 g

Saturated Fat 1 g

Cholesterol 74 mg

Sodium 209 mg

Total Carbohydrate 22 g

Dietary Fiber 3 g

Total Sugars 16 g

Protein 24 g

Potassium 655 mg

Pork with Cranberry Relish

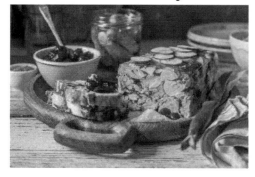

Preparation Time: 30 minutes

Cooking Time: 30 minutes

Servings: 4

Ingredients:

12 oz. pork tenderloin, fat trimmed and sliced crosswise

Salt and pepper to taste

¼ cup all-purpose flour

2 tablespoons olive oil

1 onion, sliced thinly

¼ cup dried cranberries

¼ cup low-sodium chicken broth

1 tablespoon balsamic vinegar

Directions:

Flatten each slice of pork using a mallet. In a dish, mix the salt, pepper and flour.

Dip each pork slice into the flour mixture.

Add oil to a pan over medium high heat.

Cook pork for 3 minutes per side or until golden crispy.

Transfer to a serving plate and cover with foil.

Cook the onion in the pan for 4 minutes.

Stir in the rest of the ingredients.

Simmer until the sauce has thickened.

Nutrition:

Calories 211

Total Fat 9 g

Saturated Fat 2 g

Cholesterol 53 mg

Sodium 116 mg

Total Carbohydrate 15 g

Dietary Fiber 1 g

Total Sugars 6 g

Protein 18 g

Potassium 378 mg

Irish Pork Roast

Preparation Time: 40 minutes

Cooking Time: 1 hour

Servings: 8

Ingredients:

1 ½ lb. parsnips, peeled and sliced into small pieces

1 ½ lb. carrots, sliced into small pieces

3 tablespoons olive oil, divided

2 teaspoons fresh thyme leaves, divided

Salt and pepper to taste

2 lb. pork loin roast

1 teaspoon honey

1 cup dry hard cider

Applesauce

Directions:

Preheat your oven to 400 degrees F.

Drizzle half of the oil over the parsnips and carrots.

Season with half of thyme, salt and pepper.

Arrange on a roasting pan.

Rub the pork with the remaining oil.

Season with the remaining thyme.

Season with salt and pepper.

Put it on the roasting pan on top of the vegetables.

Roast for 65 minutes.

Let cool before slicing.

Transfer the carrots and parsnips in a bowl and mix with honey.

Add the cider.

Place in a pan and simmer over low heat until the sauce has thickened.

Serve the pork with the vegetables and applesauce.

Nutrition:

Calories 272

Total Fat 8 g

Saturated Fat 2 g

Cholesterol 61 mg

Sodium 327 mg

Total Carbohydrate 23 g

Dietary Fiber 6 g

Total Sugars 10 g

Protein 24 g

Potassium 887 mg

Sesame Pork with Mustard Sauce

Preparation Time: 25 minutes

Cooking Time: 25 minutes

Servings: 4

Ingredients:

2 tablespoons low-sodium teriyaki sauce

¼ cup chili sauce

2 cloves garlic, minced

2 teaspoons ginger, grated

2 pork tenderloins

2 teaspoons sesame seeds

¼ cup low fat sour cream

1 teaspoon Dijon mustard

Salt to taste

1 scallion, chopped

Directions:

Preheat your oven to 425 degrees F.

Mix the teriyaki sauce, chili sauce, garlic and ginger.

Put the pork on a roasting pan.

Brush the sauce on both sides of the pork.

Bake in the oven for 15 minutes.

Brush with more sauce.

Top with sesame seeds.

Roast for 10 more minutes.

Mix the rest of the ingredients.

Serve the pork with mustard sauce.

Nutrition:

Calories 135

Total Fat 3 g

Saturated Fat 1 g

Cholesterol 56X mg

Sodium 302 mg

Total Carbohydrate 7 g

Dietary Fiber 1 g

Total Sugars 15 g

Protein 20 g

Potassium 755 mg

Steak with Mushroom Sauce

Preparation Time: 20 minutes

Cooking Time: 5 minutes

Servings: 4

Ingredients:

12 oz. sirloin steak, sliced and trimmed

2 teaspoons grilling seasoning

2 teaspoons oil

6 oz. broccoli, trimmed

2 cups frozen peas

3 cups fresh mushrooms, sliced

1 cup beef broth (unsalted)

1 tablespoon mustard

2 teaspoons cornstarch

Salt to taste

Directions:

Preheat your oven to 350 degrees F.

Season meat with grilling seasoning.

In a pan over medium high heat, cook the meat and broccoli for 4 minutes.

Sprinkle the peas around the steak.

Put the pan inside the oven and bake for 8 minutes.

Remove both meat and vegetables from the pan.

Add the mushrooms to the pan.

Cook for 3 minutes.

Mix the broth, mustard, salt and cornstarch.

Add to the mushrooms.

Cook for 1 minute.

Pour sauce over meat and vegetables before serving.

Nutrition:

Calories 226 - Total Fat 6 g

Saturated Fat 2 g - Cholesterol 51 mg

Sodium 356 mg

Total Carbohydrate 16 g

Dietary Fiber 5 g - Total Sugars 6 g

Protein 26 g - Potassium 780 mg

Steak with Tomato & Herbs

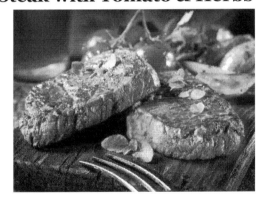

Preparation Time: 30 minutes

Cooking Time: 30 minutes

Servings: 2

Ingredients:

8 oz. beef loin steak, sliced in half

Salt and pepper to taste

Cooking spray

1 teaspoon fresh basil, snipped

¼ cup green onion, sliced

½ cup tomato, chopped

Directions:

Season the steak with salt and pepper.

Spray oil on your pan.

Put the pan over medium high heat.

Once hot, add the steaks.

Reduce heat to medium.

Cook for 10 to 13 minutes for medium, turning once.

Add the basil and green onion.

Cook for 2 minutes.

Add the tomato.

Cook for 1 minute.

Let cool a little before slicing.

Nutrition:

Calories 170 - Total Fat 6 g

Saturated Fat 2 g - Cholesterol 66 mg

Sodium 207 mg

Total Carbohydrate 3 g

Dietary Fiber 1 g - Total Sugars 5 g

Protein 25 g

Potassium 477 mg

Barbecue Beef Brisket

Preparation Time: 25 minutes

Cooking Time: 10 hours

Servings: 10

Ingredients:

4 lb. beef brisket (boneless), trimmed and sliced

1 bay leaf

2 onions, sliced into rings

½ teaspoon dried thyme, crushed

¼ cup chili sauce

1 clove garlic, minced

Salt and pepper to taste

2 tablespoons light brown sugar

2 tablespoons cornstarch

2 tablespoons cold water

Directions:

Put the meat in a slow cooker.

Add the bay leaf and onion.

In a bowl, mix the thyme, chili sauce, salt, pepper and sugar.

Pour the sauce over the meat.

Mix well.

Seal the pot and cook on low heat for 10 hours.

Discard the bay leaf.

Pour cooking liquid in a pan.

Add the mixed water and cornstarch.

Simmer until the sauce has thickened.

Pour the sauce over the meat.

Nutrition:

Calories 182

Total Fat 6 g

Saturated Fat 2 g

Cholesterol 57 mg

Sodium 217 mg

Total Carbohydrate 9 g

Dietary Fiber 1 g

Total Sugars 4 g

Protein 20 g

Potassium 383 mg

Beef & Asparagus

Preparation Time: 15 minutes

Cooking Time: 10 minutes

Servings: 4

Ingredients:

2 teaspoons olive oil

1 lb. lean beef sirloin, trimmed and sliced

1 carrot, shredded

Salt and pepper to taste

12 oz. asparagus, trimmed and sliced

1 teaspoon dried herbs de Provence, crushed

½ cup Marsala

¼ teaspoon lemon zest

Directions:

Pour oil in a pan over medium heat.

Add the beef and carrot.

Season with salt and pepper.

Cook for 3 minutes.

Add the asparagus and herbs.

Cook for 2 minutes.

Add the Marsala and lemon zest.

Cook for 5 minutes, stirring frequently.

Nutrition:

Calories 327

Total Fat 7 g

Saturated Fat 2 g

Cholesterol 69 mg

Sodium 209 mg

Total Carbohydrate 29 g

Dietary Fiber 2 g

Total Sugars 3 g

Protein 28 g

Potassium 576 mg

CHAPTER 11:

Dinner Recipes

Almond-Crusted Salmon

Preparation Time: 10 minutes

Cooking Time: 15 minutes

Servings: 4

Ingredients:

¼ cup almond meal

¼ cup whole-wheat breadcrumbs

¼ teaspoon ground coriander

1/8 teaspoon ground cumin

4 (6-ounce) boneless salmon fillets

1 tablespoon fresh lemon juice

Salt and pepper

Directions:

Preheat the oven to 500°F and line a small baking dish with foil.

Combine the almond meal, breadcrumbs, coriander, and cumin in a small bowl. Rinse the fish in cool water then pat dry and brush with lemon juice. Season the fish with salt and pepper then dredge in the almond mixture on both sides. Place the fish in the baking dish and bake for 15 minutes until it just flakes with a fork.

Nutrition:

Calories 295 - Fat 14.3g

Saturated Fat 1.9g

Total Carbs 6.5g - Net Carbs 5.4g

Protein 35.5g - Sugar 0.5g

Fiber 1.1g - Sodium 128mg

Chicken & Veggie Bowl with Brown Rice

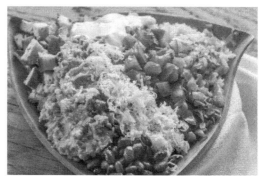

Preparation Time: 10 minutes

Cooking Time: 20 minutes

Servings: 4

Ingredients:

1 cup instant brown rice

¼ cup tahini

¼ cup fresh lemon juice

2 cloves minced garlic

¼ teaspoon ground cumin

Pinch salt

1 tablespoon olive oil

4 (4-ounce) chicken breast halves

½ medium yellow onion, sliced

1 cup green beans, trimmed

1 cup chopped broccoli

4 cups chopped kale

Directions:

Bring 1 cup water to boil in a small saucepan.

Stir in the brown rice and simmer for 5 minutes then cover and set aside.

Meanwhile, whisk together the tahini with ¼ cup water in a small bowl.

Stir in the lemon juice, garlic, and cumin with a pinch of salt and stir well.

Heat the oil in a large cast-iron skillet over medium heat.

Season the chicken with salt and pepper then add to the skillet.

Cook for 3 to 5 minutes on each side until cooked through then remove to a cutting board and cover loosely with foil.

Reheat the skillet and cook the onion for 2 minutes then stir in the broccoli and beans.

Sauté for 2 minutes then stir in the kale and sauté 2 minutes more.

Add 2 tablespoons of water then cover and steam for 2 minutes while you slice the chicken.

Build the bowls with brown rice, sliced chicken, and sautéed veggies.

Serve hot drizzled with the lemon tahini dressing.

Nutrition:

Calories 435

Fat 20.5g

Saturated Fat 4.1g

Total Carbs 24.1g

Net Carbs 19.3g

Protein 39.9g

Sugar 1.8g

Fiber 4.8g

Sodium 196mg

Beef Fajitas

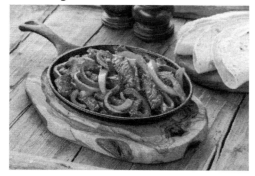

Preparation Time: 10 minutes

Cooking Time: 15 minutes

Servings: 4

Ingredients:

1 lbs. lean beef sirloin, sliced thin

1 tablespoon olive oil

1 medium red onion, sliced

1 red pepper, sliced thin

1 green pepper, sliced thin

½ teaspoon ground cumin

½ teaspoon chili powder

8 (6-inch) whole-wheat tortillas

Fat-free sour cream

Directions:

Heat a large cast-iron skillet over medium heat then add the oil.

Add the sliced beef and cook in a single layer for 1 minute on each side.

Remove the beef to a bowl and cover to keep warm.

Reheat the skillet then add the onions and peppers – season with cumin and chili powder.

Stir-fry the veggies to your liking then add to the bowl with the beef.

Serve hot in small whole-wheat tortillas with sliced avocado and fat-free sour cream.

Nutrition:

Calories 430

Fat 14.8g

Saturated Fat 3.2g

Total Carbs 30.5g

Net Carbs 12.9g

Protein 41.2g

Sugar 3.4g

Fiber 17.6g

Sodium 561mg

Sautéed Turkey Bowl

Preparation Time: 20 minutes

Cooking Time: 10 minutes

Servings: 1

Ingredients:

4 ounces boneless, skinless turkey breast

1 teaspoon olive oil

1 ½ teaspoons balsamic vinegar

½ teaspoon dried basil

¼ teaspoon dried thyme

Salt and pepper

¼ cup instant brown rice

Directions:

Toss the turkey with the olive oil, balsamic vinegar, basil, and thyme.

Season lightly with salt and pepper then cover and chill for 20 minutes.

Bring ¼ cup of water to boil in a small saucepan. Stir in the brown rice then simmer for 5 minutes and remove from heat, covered.

Meanwhile, heat a small skillet over medium heat and grease lightly with cooking spray. Add the marinated turkey and sauté for 6 to 8 minutes until cooked through.

Spoon the turkey over the brown rice and serve hot.

Nutrition:

Calories 200

Fat 6.8g

Saturated Fat 1.1g

Total Carbs 13.3g

Net Carbs 12.1g

Protein 20.4g

Sugar 4g

Fiber 1.2g

Sodium 1152mg

Chicken Mushroom Stroganoff

Preparation Time: 5 minutes

Cooking Time: 25 minutes

Servings: 6

Ingredients:

1 cup fat-free sour cream

2 tablespoons flour

1 tablespoon Worcestershire sauce

½ teaspoon dried thyme

1 chicken bouillon cube, crushed

Salt and pepper

½ cup water

1 medium yellow onion, chopped

8 ounces sliced mushrooms

1 tablespoon olive oil

2 cloves minced garlic

12 ounces boneless skinless chicken breast, cooked and shredded

6 ounces whole-wheat noodles, cooked

Directions:

Whisk together 2/3 cup of the sour cream with the flour, Worcestershire sauce, thyme, and crushed bouillon in a medium bowl.

Season with salt and pepper then slowly stir in the water until well combined.

Heat the oil in a large skillet over medium-high heat.

Add the onions and mushrooms and sauté for 3 minutes.

Stir in the garlic and cook for 2 minutes more then add the chicken.

Pour in the sour cream mixture and cook until thick and bubbling.

Reduce heat and simmer for 2 minutes.

Spoon the chicken and mushroom mixture over the cooked noodles and garnish with the remaining sour cream to serve.

Nutrition:

Calories 295 - Fat 7.8g

Saturated Fat 2g - Total Carbs 29.6g

Net Carbs 26.7g

Protein 24.6g - Sugar 4.7g

Fiber 2.9g - Sodium 225mg

Grilled Tuna Kebabs

Preparation Time: 20 minutes

Cooking Time: 10 minutes

Servings: 4

Ingredients:

2 ½ tablespoons rice vinegar

2 tablespoons fresh grated ginger

2 tablespoons sesame oil

2 tablespoons soy sauce

2 tablespoons fresh chopped cilantro

1 tablespoon minced green chili

1 ½ pounds fresh ahi tuna, cut into 1 ¼-inch cubes

1 large red pepper, cut into 1-inch pieces

1 large red onion, cut into 1-inch pieces

Directions:

Whisk together the rice vinegar, ginger, sesame oil, soy sauce, cilantro, and chili in a medium bowl – add a few drops of liquid stevia extract to sweeten.

Toss in the tuna and chill for 20 minutes covered.

Meanwhile, grease a grill pan with cooking spray and soak wooden skewers in water.

Slide the tuna cubes onto the skewers with red pepper and onion.

Grill for 3 to 4 minutes on each side until done to your liking and serve hot.

Nutrition:

Calories 240 - Fat 8.2g

Saturated Fat 1g - Total Carbs 8.5g

Net Carbs 6.8g - Protein 31.5g

Sugar 3.4g

Fiber 1.7g

Sodium 503mg

Cast-Iron Pork Loin

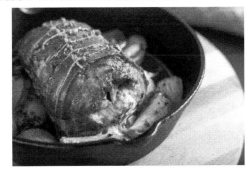

Preparation Time: 10 minutes

Cooking Time: 20 minutes

Servings: 6

Ingredients:

1 (1 ½ pounds) boneless pork loin

Salt and pepper

2 tablespoons olive oil

2 tablespoons dried herb blend

Directions:

Heat the oven to 425°F.

Trim the excess fat from the pork and season with salt and pepper.

Heat the oil in a large cast-iron skillet over medium heat.

Add the pork and cook for 2 minutes on each side.

Sprinkle the herbs over the pork and transfer to the oven.

Roast for 10 to 15 minutes until the internal temperature reaches 145°F.

Remove to a cutting board and let rest 5 to 10 minutes before slicing to serve.

Nutrition:

Calories 205

Fat 8.7g

Saturated Fat 2g

Total Carbs 1g

Net Carbs 1g

Protein 29.8g

Sugar 0g

Fiber 0g

Sodium 65mg

Crispy Baked Tofu

Preparation Time: 5 minutes

Cooking Time: 25 minutes

Servings: 4

Ingredients:

1 (14-ounce) block extra-firm tofu

1 tablespoon olive oil

1 tablespoon cornstarch

½ teaspoon garlic powder

Salt and pepper

Directions:

Lay some paper towels out on a flat surface.

Cut the tofu into slices up to about ½-inch thick and lay them out.

Cover the tofu with another paper towel and place a cutting board on top.

Let the tofu drain for 10 to 15 minutes.

Preheat the oven to 400°F and line a baking sheet with foil or parchment.

Cut the tofu into cubes and place in a large bowl.

Toss with the olive oil, cornstarch, garlic powder, salt and pepper until coated.

Spread on the baking sheet and bake for 10 minutes.

Flip the tofu and bake for another 10 to 15 minutes until crisp. Serve hot.

Nutrition:

Calories 140

Fat 8.7g

Saturated Fat 1.1g

Total Carbs 2.1g

Net Carbs 2g

Protein 12.7g

Sugar 0.1g

Fiber 0.1g

Sodium 23mg

Tilapia with Coconut Rice

Preparation Time: 10 minutes

Cooking Time: 15 minutes

Servings: 4

Ingredients:

4 (6-ounce) boneless tilapia fillets

1 tablespoon ground turmeric

Salt and pepper

1 tablespoon olive oil

2 (8.8-ounce) packets precooked whole-grain rice

1 cup light coconut milk, shaken

½ cup fresh chopped cilantro

1 ½ tablespoons fresh lime juice

Directions:

Season the fish with turmeric, salt, and pepper.

Heat the oil in a large skillet over medium heat and add the fish.

Cook for 2 to 3 minutes per side until golden brown.

Remove the fish to a plate and cover to keep warm.

Reheat the skillet and add the rice, coconut milk, and a pinch of salt.

Simmer on high heat until thickened, about 3 to 4 minutes.

Stir in the cilantro and lime juice.

Spoon the rice onto plates and serve with the cooked fish.

Nutrition:

Calories 460

Fat 25.2g

Saturated Fat 15.3g

Total Carbs 27.1g

Net Carbs 23.4g

Protein 34.8g

Sugar 2.4g

Fiber 3.7g

Sodium 145mg

Spicy Turkey Tacos

Preparation Time: 5 minutes

Cooking Time: 25 minutes

Servings: 8

Ingredients:

1 tablespoon olive oil

1 medium yellow onion, diced

2 cloves minced garlic

1 pound 93% lean ground turkey

1 cup tomato sauce, no sugar added

1 jalapeno, seeded and minced

8 low-carb multigrain tortillas

Directions:

Heat the oil in a large skillet over medium heat. Add the onion and sauté for 4 minutes then stir in the garlic and cook 1 minute more. Stir in the ground turkey and cook for 5 minutes until browned, breaking it up with a wooden spoon.

Sprinkle on the taco seasoning and cayenne then stir well. Cook for 30 seconds then stir in the tomato sauce and jalapeno. Simmer on low heat for 10 minutes while you warm the tortillas in the microwave. Serve the meat in the tortillas with your favorite taco toppings.

Nutrition:

Calories 195

Fat 7.8g

Saturated Fat 1.5g

Total Carbs 15.4g

Net Carbs 7.4g

Protein 14.2g

Sugar 1.6g

Fiber 8g

Sodium 380mg

Quick and Easy Shrimp Stir-Fry

Preparation Time: 15 minutes

Cooking Time: 15 minutes

Servings: 5

Ingredients:

1 tablespoon olive oil

1-pound uncooked shrimp, peeled and deveined

Salt and pepper

1 tablespoon sesame oil

8 ounces snow peas

4 ounces broccoli, chopped

1 medium red pepper, sliced

3 cloves minced garlic

1 tablespoon fresh grated ginger

½ cup soy sauce

1 tablespoon cornstarch

2 tablespoons fresh lime juice

¼ teaspoon liquid stevia extract

Directions:

Heat the olive oil in a large skillet over medium heat.

Add the shrimp and season with salt and pepper then sauté until just pink, about 5 minutes.

Remove the shrimp to a bowl and keep warm.

Reheat the skillet with the sesame oil and add the veggies.

Sauté until the veggies are tender, about 6 to 8 minutes.

Stir in the garlic and ginger and cook for 1 minute more.

Whisk together the remaining ingredients and pour into the skillet.

Toss to coat the veggies then add the shrimp and reheat. Serve hot.

Nutrition:

Calories 220

Fat 7.4g

Saturated Fat 1.3g

Total Carbs 12.7g

Net Carbs 10.1g

Protein 24.8g

Sugar 3.9g

Fiber 2.6g

Sodium 1670mg

Chicken Burrito Bowl with Quinoa

Preparation Time: 15 minutes

Cooking Time: 10 minutes

Servings: 6

Ingredients:

1 tablespoon chipotle chiles in adobo, chopped

1 tablespoon olive oil

½ teaspoon garlic powder

½ teaspoon ground cumin

1-pound boneless skinless chicken breast

Salt and pepper

2 cups cooked quinoa

2 cups shredded romaine lettuce

1 cup black beans, rinsed and drained

1 cup diced avocado

3 tablespoons fat-free sour cream

Directions:

Stir together the chipotle chiles, olive oil, garlic powder, and cumin in a small bowl.

Preheat a grill pan to medium-high and grease with cooking spray.

Season the chicken with salt and pepper and add to the grill pan.

Grill for 5 minutes then flip it and brush with the chipotle glaze.

Cook for another 3 to 5 minutes until cooked through.

Remove to a cutting board and chop the chicken.

Assemble the bowls with 1/6 of the quinoa, chicken, lettuce, beans, and avocado.

Top each with a half tablespoon of fat-free sour cream to serve.

Nutrition:

Calories 410

Fat 14.7g

Saturated Fat 3g

Total Carbs 37.4g

Net Carbs 28.9g

Protein 32.4g

Sugar 1.6g

Fiber 8.5g

Sodium 97mg

Baked Salmon Cakes

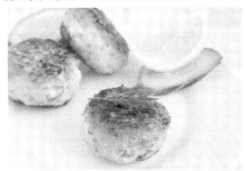

Preparation Time: 10 minutes

Cooking Time: 20 minutes

Servings: 4

Ingredients:

15 ounces canned salmon, drained

1 large egg

whisked

2 teaspoons Dijon mustard

1 small yellow onion, minced

1 ½ cups whole-wheat breadcrumbs

¼ cup low-fat mayonnaise

¼ cup nonfat Greek yogurt, plain

1 tablespoon fresh chopped parsley

1 tablespoon fresh lemon juice

2 green onions, sliced thin

Directions:

Preheat the oven to 450°F and line a baking sheet with parchment.

Flake the salmon into a medium bowl then stir in the egg and mustard.

Mix in the onions and breadcrumbs by hand, blending well, then shape into 8 patties.

Grease a large skillet and heat it over medium heat.

Add the patties and fry for 2 minutes on each side until browned.

Transfer the patties to the baking sheet and bake for 15 minutes or until cooked through.

Meanwhile, whisk together the remaining ingredients.

Serve the baked salmon cakes with the creamy herb sauce.

Nutrition:

Calories 240

Fat 12.2g

Saturated Fat 1.4g

Total Carbs 9.3g

Net Carbs 7.8g

Protein 25g

Sugar 1.8g

Fiber 1.5g

Sodium 241mg

CHAPTER 12:

Vegetables

Arugula and Chorizo Salad Recipe

Preparation Time: 18 minutes

Cooking Time: 20 minutes

Servings: 4

Ingredients:

Rosemary, chopped 1 tablespoon

Garlic (minced): cloves

Salt and black pepper

Chorizo sausage (sliced): 1

Arugula: 4 cups

Olive oil: 1 tablespoon

Green onions (chopped): 2

For the salad covering:

Apple vinegar: 2 tablespoons

Lemon juice: ½ teaspoon

Mustard: 2 teaspoons

Olive oil: 4 tablespoons

Directions:

Heat a pan with 1 tablespoon of oil over medium heat, add garlic, rosemary, salt, and pepper, stir and cook for 5 minutes. Add chorizo, stir, cook for 3 minutes, put everything in a salad bowl, add rocket and spring onions and dice. Mix 4 tablespoons of oil with lemon juice, vinegar, mustard and black pepper in a bowl, beat well, add the salad, toss and serve. Enjoy!

Nutrition:

fat 6 - fiber 6 - calories 176

carbs 6 - protein 7

Avocado n Egg Salad

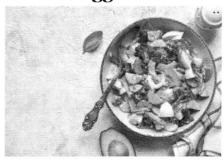

Preparation Time: 21 minutes

Servings: 3

Ingredients:

Avocado-1 (pitted, peeled and cut into chunks)

Homemade mayonnaise 1/4 cup

Eggs-6

Mustard-1 teaspoon

Lemon juice-1 teaspoon

Dill-1 teaspoon (chopped)

Parsley-1/2 tablespoon (chopped)

Salt and black pepper-A pinch

Directions:

Beat in the eggs in a pot. Cover them with water. Bring to a simmer. Cook them for 10 minutes. Drain and rinse them with cold water. Peel, chop and put them in a salad bowl. Add mayonnaise, avocado, mustard, lemon juice, parsley, dill, salt and pepper. Stir well and serve for lunch. Enjoy!

Nutrition:

calories 206 - fat 6

fiber 6 - carbs 16

protein 6

Broccoli Stew with lemon flavor

Preparation Time: 30 minutes

Cooking Time: 20 minutes

Servings: 2

Ingredients:

Two chopped tomatoes

Chopped red onion - ½ cup

lemon juice - 1 teaspoon

veggie stock - 2 cups

Coriander (ground) - 1 teaspoon

Minced garlic cloves- Four

Broccoli florets - 1 cup

Cumin seeds - ½ teaspoon

Turmeric powder- ½ teaspoon

Seasoning- A pinch of salt and black pepper

Olive oil - ½ teaspoon

Directions:

Mix tomatoes with garlic, onion, salt, pepper, coriander, and turmeric in a blender and pulse really well.

With medium temperature, heat up a pan with the oil, add tomato, stir and sauté for ten minutes.

Put cumin, broccoli, stock, and lemon juice, mix well, cook for 10 minutes.

Divide into separate bowls and serve.

Enjoy!

Nutrition:

calories 196

fat 6

fiber 6

carbs 16

protein 8

Brussels Sprouts Soup with chicken stock

Preparation Time: 30 minutes

Cooking Time: 20 minutes

Servings: 4

Ingredients:

Brussels sprouts (trimmed and halved): 2 pounds

A pinch of salt and black pepper

Yellow onion (chopped): 1

Olive oil: 2 tablespoons

Chicken stock: 4 cups

Coconut cream: ¼ cup

Directions:

Heat a pan with the oil over medium heat, add the onion, stir and cook for 3 minutes.

Add Brussels sprouts, broth, salt, and pepper stir, simmer and cook for 20 minutes. Use a hand blender to make your cream, add cream, stir, shovel into bowls and serve.

Enjoy!

Nutrition:

calories 196

fiber 6

carbs 6

fat 16

protein 8

Buttered Asparagus

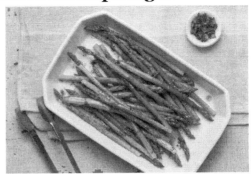

Preparation Time: 25 minutes

Cooking Time: 15

Servings: 4

Ingredients:

Medium eggs, 4

Butter, 5 oz.

Avocado oil, 1 tbsp.

Cayenne pepper, ¼ tsp.

Sour cream, 8 tbsps.

Salt

Trimmed asparagus, 1½ lbs.

Black pepper

Grated Parmesan cheese, 3 oz.

Lemon juice, 1 ½ tbsps.

Directions:

Set the pan over medium-high heat to melt 2 oz. butter.

Stir in the seasoning and eggs.

Set your blender in position, add in the eggs, sour cream, seasonings, parmesan cheese, and cayenne pepper. Blend until well combined.

Set the pan over medium-high heat to roast the asparagus with the seasonings. Reserve in a plate.

Set the same pan again over medium-high heat to brown the rest of butter

Remove from heat then stir in the lemon juice

Melt the butter again then set the asparagus to the pan to coat evenly

Heat then divide on plates topped with blended eggs

Nutrition:

Calories: 566

Fat: 46

Fiber: 16

Carbs: 26

Protein: 22

Butternut Squash Salad

Preparation Time: 10 minutes

Cooking Time: 0

Servings: 2

Ingredients:

Walnuts (chopped): 1/3 cup

Salt and black pepper

Butternut squash (baked, peeled and cut into wedges): 10 oz

Olive oil: 2 tablespoons

White vinegar: 1 tablespoon

Mustard: ½ teaspoon

Lettuce leaves (torn): 3 cups

Cinnamon powder: ¼ teaspoon

Directions:

Mix the pumpkin in a bowl with vinegar, walnuts, cinnamon, oil, mustard, lettuce, salt and pepper and serve.

Enjoy!

Nutrition:

calories 126

fat 6

carbs 6

fiber 6

protein 11

Cabbage and Brussels Sprouts Salad

Preparation Time: 10 minutes

Cooking Time: 0

Servings: 4

Ingredients:

Red cabbage (chopped): 2 cups

Brussels sprouts (shredded): 4 cups

Salt and black pepper

Walnuts (chopped): ¼ cup

Lemon juice: 2 tablespoons

Balsamic vinegar: 4 tablespoons

Avocado mayonnaise: ¼ cup

Directions:

In a salad bowl, combine the cabbage with Brussels sprouts, walnuts, salt, pepper, vinegar, mayo and lemon juice, dice and serve.

Enjoy!

Nutrition:

calories 90

fiber 1

fat 0

carbs 6

protein 7

Cabbage with Coconut aminos Salad

Preparation Time: 10 minutes

Cooking Time: 0

Servings: 4

Ingredients:

Avocado mayonnaise: ½ cup

Lime juice: 1 teaspoon

Salt and black pepper

Stevia: 1 teaspoon

Fennel bulb (sliced): 1

Coconut aminos: 1 and ½ teaspoons

Red cabbage head (sliced): 1

Parsley (chopped): 1 bunch

Directions:

Mix the fennel in a salad bowl with cabbage, parsley, salt, and pepper.

Add coconut aminos, mayonnaise, lime juice, and stevia shake well and serve.

Enjoy!

Nutrition:

fat 6

fiber 6

carbs 6

calories 186

protein 11

Capers Eggplant Medley

Preparation Time: 40 minutes

Cooking Time: 0

Servings: 4

Ingredients:

Eggplants; cut into medium chunks 2

Red onion; chopped-1

Oregano; dried-1 teaspoon

Olive oil-2 tablespoons

Capers; chopped-2 tablespoons

Garlic cloves; chopped-2

Parsley; a chopped-1 bunch

Green olives; pitted and sliced-1 handful

Tomatoes; chopped-5

Herb vinegar-3 tablespoons

Salt and black pepper -to the taste.

Directions:

Add a cooking pot with cooking oil on medium heat. Toss in eggplants along with salt, pepper, and oregano. Stir cook for 5 minutes then add parsley, onion, and garlic. Sauté for 4 minutes then add tomatoes, vinegar, olives, and capers. Cook for 15 minutes then adjust seasoning with salt and pepper.

Enjoy fresh.

Nutrition:

Calories: 200;

Fat: 1g

Fiber: g

Carbs: g

Protein: 7g

Swiss Vegetable Soup

Preparation Time: 2 hours 20 minutes

Cooking Time: 0

Servings: 4

Ingredients:

Red onion; chopped-1

Swiss chard; a chopped-1 bunch

Yellow squash; chopped-1

Zucchini; chopped-1

Green bell pepper; chopped-1

Sausage; chopped-1 pound

Garlic cloves; minced-2

Cauliflower florets; chopped-1 cup

Green beans; chopped-1 cup

Chicken stock-6 cups

Canned tomato paste-7 ounces

Water-2 cups

Thyme; chopped-2 teaspoons

Rosemary; dried-1 teaspoon

Fennel; minced-1 tablespoon

Red pepper flakes 1/2 teaspoon

Some grated parmesan for serving

Carrots; chopped-6

Tomatoes; chopped-4 cups

Salt and black pepper -to the taste

Directions:

Place a skillet over medium-high heat.

Add garlic and sausage, sauté until brown then transfer to a slow cooker.

Add squash, onion, bell pepper, Swiss chard, carrots, tomatoes, green beans, zucchini, cauliflower, water, stock, tomato paste, fennel, rosemary, salt, pepper, and pepper flakes.

Cover the mixture in the slow cooker and cook on High for 2 hours.

Remove the lid from the cooker and mix well.

Drizzle parmesan cheese and serve right away.

Nutrition:

Calories: 150;

Fat: 7

Fiber: 8

Carbs: 21

Protein: 9g

CHAPTER 13:

Meat Recipes

Pork Chops with Grape Sauce

Preparation Time: 15 minutes

Cooking Time: 25 minutes

Servings: 4

Ingredients:

Cooking spray

4 pork chops

¼ cup onion, sliced

1 clove garlic, minced

½ cup low-sodium chicken broth

¾ cup apple juice

1 tablespoon cornstarch

1 tablespoon balsamic vinegar

1 teaspoon honey

1 cup seedless red grapes, sliced in half

Directions:

Spray oil on your pan.

Put it over medium heat.

Add the pork chops to the pan.

Cook for 5 minutes per side.

Remove and set aside.

Add onion and garlic.

Cook for 2 minutes.

Pour in the broth and apple juice.

Bring to a boil.

Reduce heat to simmer. Put the pork chops back to the skillet. Simmer for 4 minutes. In a bowl, mix the cornstarch, vinegar and honey. Add to the pan. Cook until the sauce has thickened.

Add the grapes. Pour sauce over the pork chops before serving.

Nutrition:

Calories 188

Total Fat 4 g

Saturated Fat 1 g

Cholesterol 47 mg

Sodium 117 mg

Total Carbohydrate 18 g

Dietary Fiber 1 g

Total Sugars 13 g

Protein 19 g

Potassium 759 mg

Roasted Pork & Apples

Preparation Time: 15 minutes

Cooking Time: 30 minutes

Servings: 4

Ingredients:

Salt and pepper to taste

½ teaspoon dried, crushed

1 lb. pork tenderloin

1 tablespoon canola oil

1 onion, sliced into wedges

3 cooking apples, sliced into wedges

⅔ cup apple cider

Sprigs fresh sage

Directions:

In a bowl, mix salt, pepper and sage.

Season both sides of pork with this mixture.

Place a pan over medium heat.

Brown both sides.

Transfer to a roasting pan.

Add the onion on top and around the pork.

Drizzle oil on top of the pork and apples.

Roast in the oven at 425 degrees F for 10 minutes.

Add the apples, roast for another 15 minutes.

In a pan, boil the apple cider and then simmer for 10 minutes.

Pour the apple cider sauce over the pork before serving.

Nutrition:

Calories 239

Total Fat 6 g

Saturated Fat 1 g

Cholesterol 74 mg

Sodium 209 mg

Total Carbohydrate 22 g

Dietary Fiber 3 g

Total Sugars 16 g

Protein 24 g

Potassium 655 mg

Pork with Cranberry Relish

Preparation Time: 30 minutes

Cooking Time: 30 minutes

Servings: 4

Ingredients:

12 oz. pork tenderloin, fat trimmed and sliced crosswise

Salt and pepper to taste

¼ cup all-purpose flour

2 tablespoons olive oil

1 onion, sliced thinly

¼ cup dried cranberries

¼ cup low-sodium chicken broth

1 tablespoon balsamic vinegar

Directions:

Flatten each slice of pork using a mallet.

In a dish, mix the salt, pepper and flour.

Dip each pork slice into the flour mixture.

Add oil to a pan over medium high heat.

Cook pork for 3 minutes per side or until golden crispy.

Transfer to a serving plate and cover with foil. Cook the onion in the pan for 4 minutes.

Stir in the rest of the ingredients.

Simmer until the sauce has thickened.

Nutrition:

Calories 211

Total Fat 9 g

Saturated Fat 2 g

Cholesterol 53 mg

Sodium 116 mg

Total Carbohydrate 15 g

Dietary Fiber 1 g

Total Sugars 6 g

Protein 18 g

Potassium 378 mg

Irish Pork Roast

Preparation Time: 40 minutes

Cooking Time: 1 hour

Servings: 8

Ingredients:

1 ½ lb. parsnips, peeled and sliced into small pieces

1 ½ lb. carrots, sliced into small pieces

3 tablespoons olive oil, divided

2 teaspoons fresh thyme leaves, divided

Salt and pepper to taste

2 lb. pork loin roast

1 teaspoon honey

1 cup dry hard cider

Applesauce

Directions:

Preheat your oven to 400 degrees F.

Drizzle half of the oil over the parsnips and carrots.

Season with half of thyme, salt and pepper.

Arrange on a roasting pan.

Rub the pork with the remaining oil.

Season with the remaining thyme.

Season with salt and pepper.

Put it on the roasting pan on top of the vegetables.

Roast for 65 minutes.

Let cool before slicing. Transfer the carrots and parsnips in a bowl and mix with honey.

Add the cider. Place in a pan and simmer over low heat until the sauce has thickened.

Serve the pork with the vegetables and applesauce.

Nutrition:

Calories 272 - Total Fat 8 g

Saturated Fat 2 g

Cholesterol 61 mg - Sodium 327 mg

Total Carbohydrate 23 g

Dietary Fiber 6 g

Total Sugars 10 g

Protein 24 g

Potassium 887 mg

Sesame Pork with Mustard Sauce

Preparation Time: 25 minutes

Cooking Time: 25 minutes

Servings: 4

Ingredients:

2 tablespoons low-sodium teriyaki sauce

¼ cup chili sauce

2 cloves garlic, minced

2 teaspoons ginger, grated

2 pork tenderloins

2 teaspoons sesame seeds

¼ cup low fat sour cream

1 teaspoon Dijon mustard

Salt to taste

1 scallion, chopped

Directions:

Preheat your oven to 425 degrees F.

Mix the teriyaki sauce, chili sauce, garlic and ginger. Put the pork on a roasting pan.

Brush the sauce on both sides of the pork. Bake in the oven for 15 minutes.

Brush with more sauce. Top with sesame seeds. Roast for 10 more minutes. Mix the rest of the ingredients.

Serve the pork with mustard sauce.

Nutrition:

Calories 135

Total Fat 3 g

Saturated Fat 1 g

Cholesterol 56X mg

Sodium 302 mg

Total Carbohydrate 7 g

Dietary Fiber 1 g

Total Sugars 15 g

Protein 20 g

Potassium 755 mg

Steak with Mushroom Sauce

Preparation Time: 20 minutes

Cooking Time: 5 minutes

Servings: 4

Ingredients:

12 oz. sirloin steak, sliced and trimmed

2 teaspoons grilling seasoning

2 teaspoons oil

6 oz. broccoli, trimmed

2 cups frozen peas

3 cups fresh mushrooms, sliced

1 cup beef broth (unsalted)

1 tablespoon mustard

2 teaspoons cornstarch

Salt to taste

Directions:

Preheat your oven to 350 degrees F.

Season meat with grilling seasoning.

In a pan over medium high heat, cook the meat and broccoli for 4 minutes.

Sprinkle the peas around the steak.

Put the pan inside the oven and bake for 8 minutes.

Remove both meat and vegetables from the pan.

Add the mushrooms to the pan.

Cook for 3 minutes.

Mix the broth, mustard, salt and cornstarch.

Add to the mushrooms.

Cook for 1 minute.

Pour sauce over meat and vegetables before serving.

Nutrition:

Calories 226

Total Fat 6 g

Saturated Fat 2 g

Cholesterol 51 mg

Sodium 356 mg

Total Carbohydrate 16 g

Dietary Fiber 5 g

Total Sugars 6 g

Protein 26 g

Potassium 780 mg

Steak with Tomato & Herbs

Preparation Time: 30 minutes

Cooking Time: 30 minutes

Servings: 2

Ingredients:

8 oz. beef loin steak, sliced in half

Salt and pepper to taste

Cooking spray

1 teaspoon fresh basil, snipped

¼ cup green onion, sliced

½ cup tomato, chopped

Directions:

Season the steak with salt and pepper.

Spray oil on your pan.

Put the pan over medium high heat.

Once hot, add the steaks.

Reduce heat to medium.

Cook for 10 to 13 minutes for medium, turning once.

Add the basil and green onion.

Cook for 2 minutes.

Add the tomato.

Cook for 1 minute.

Let cool a little before slicing.

Nutrition:

Calories 170

Total Fat 6 g

Saturated Fat 2 g

Cholesterol 66 mg

Sodium 207 mg

Total Carbohydrate 3 g

Dietary Fiber 1 g

Total Sugars 5 g

Protein 25 g

Potassium 477 mg

Barbecue Beef Brisket

Preparation Time: 25 minutes

Cooking Time: 10 hours

Servings: 10

Ingredients:

4 lb. beef brisket (boneless), trimmed and sliced

1 bay leaf

2 onions, sliced into rings

½ teaspoon dried thyme, crushed

¼ cup chili sauce

1 clove garlic, minced

Salt and pepper to taste

2 tablespoons light brown sugar

2 tablespoons cornstarch

2 tablespoons cold water

Directions:

Put the meat in a slow cooker.

Add the bay leaf and onion.

In a bowl, mix the thyme, chili sauce, salt, pepper and sugar.

Pour the sauce over the meat.

Mix well.

Seal the pot and cook on low heat for 10 hours.

Discard the bay leaf.

Pour cooking liquid in a pan.

Add the mixed water and cornstarch.

Simmer until the sauce has thickened.

Pour the sauce over the meat.

Nutrition:

Calories 182

Total Fat 6 g

Saturated Fat 2 g

Cholesterol 57 mg

Sodium 217 mg

Total Carbohydrate 9 g

Dietary Fiber 1 g

Total Sugars 4 g

Protein 20 g

Potassium 383 mg

Beef & Asparagus

Preparation Time: 15 minutes

Cooking Time: 10 minutes

Servings: 4

Ingredients:

2 teaspoons olive oil

1 lb. lean beef sirloin, trimmed and sliced

1 carrot, shredded

Salt and pepper to taste

12 oz. asparagus, trimmed and sliced

1 teaspoon dried herbs de Provence, crushed

½ cup Marsala

¼ teaspoon lemon zest

Directions:

Pour oil in a pan over medium heat.

Add the beef and carrot.

Season with salt and pepper.

Cook for 3 minutes.

Add the asparagus and herbs.

Cook for 2 minutes.

Add the Marsala and lemon zest.

Cook for 5 minutes, stirring frequently.

Nutrition:

Calories 327

Total Fat 7 g

Saturated Fat 2 g

Cholesterol 69 mg

Sodium 209 mg

Total Carbohydrate 29 g

Dietary Fiber 2 g

Total Sugars 3 g

Protein 28 g

Potassium 576 mg

CHAPTER 14:

Snacks

Cinnamon Spiced Popcorn

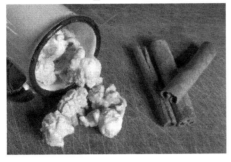

Preparation Time: 10 minutes

Cooking Time: 5 minutes

Servings: 4

Ingredients:

8 cups air-popped corn

2 teaspoons sugar

½ to 1 teaspoon ground cinnamon

Butter-flavored cooking spray

Directions:

Preheat the oven to 350°F and line a shallow roasting pan with foil.

Pop the popcorn using your preferred method.

Spread the popcorn in the roasting pan and mix the sugar and cinnamon in a small bowl.

Lightly spray the popcorn with cooking spray and toss to coat evenly.

Sprinkle with cinnamon and toss again.

Bake for 5 minutes until just crisp then serve warm.

Nutrition:

Calories 70

Fat 0.7g

Saturated Fat 0.1g

Total Carbs 14.7g

Net Carbs 12.2g

Protein 2.1g

Sugar 2.2g

Fiber 2.5g

Sodium 1mg

Grilled Peaches

Preparation Time: 5 minutes

Cooking Time: 10 minutes

Servings: 6

Ingredients:

6 fresh peaches, ripe

1 tablespoon olive oil

6 tablespoons fat-free whipped topping

Directions:

Lightly grease a grill pan and preheat it over medium heat. Cut the peaches in half and remove the pits. Brush the cut sides with olive oil or spritz with cooking spray. Place the peaches cut side down on the grill for 4 to 5 minutes. Flip the peaches and cook for another 4 to 5 minutes until tender. Spoon the peaches into bowls and serve with fat-free whipped topping.

Nutrition:

Calories 100 - Fat 2.7g

Saturated Fat 0.3g

Total Carbs 18g

Net Carbs 15.7g

Protein 1.4g

Sugar 16g

Fiber 2.3g

Sodium 10mg

Peanut Butter Banana "Ice Cream"

Preparation Time: 10 minutes

Cooking Time: 0 minutes

Servings: 6

Ingredients:

4 medium bananas

½ cup whipped peanut butter

1 teaspoon vanilla extract

Directions:

Peel the bananas and slice them into coins. Arrange the slices on a plate and freeze until solid. Place the frozen bananas in a food processor. Add the peanut butter and pulse until it is mostly smooth. Scrape down the sides then add the vanilla extract. Pulse until smooth then spoon into bowls to serve.

Nutrition:

Calories 165

Fat 8.3g

Saturated Fat 1.8g

Total Carbs 21.4g

Net Carbs 18g

Protein 4.9g

Sugar 11g

Fiber 3.4g

Sodium 74mg

Fruity Coconut Energy Balls

Preparation Time: 15 minutes

Cooking Time: 0 minutes

Servings: 18

Ingredients:

1 cup chopped almonds

1 cup dried figs

½ cup dried apricots, chopped

½ cup dried cranberries, unsweetened

½ teaspoon vanilla extract

¼ teaspoon ground cinnamon

½ cup shredded unsweetened coconut

Directions:

Place the almonds, figs, apricots, and cranberries in a food processor. Pulse the mixture until finely chopped. Add the vanilla extract and cinnamon then pulse to combine once more. Roll the mixture into 18 small balls by hand. Roll the balls in the shredded coconut and chill until firm.

Nutrition:

Calories 100 - Fat 4.9g

Saturated Fat 2.1g

Total Carbs 14.6g

Net Carbs 11.9g - Protein 1.8g

Sugar 10.7g

Fiber 2.7g

Sodium 3mg

Strawberry Salsa

Preparation Time: 10 minutes

Cooking Time: 5 minutes

Servings: 4

Ingredients:

4 tomatoes, seeded and chopped

1-pint strawberry, chopped

1 red onion, chopped

2 tablespoons of juice from a lime

1 jalapeno pepper, minced

What you will need from the store cupboard:

1 tablespoon olive oil

2 garlic cloves, minced

Instructions:

Bring together the strawberries, tomatoes, jalapeno, and onion in the bowl. Stir in the garlic, oil, and lime juice. Refrigerate. Serve with separately cooked pork or poultry.

Nutrition:

Calories 19,

Carbohydrates 3g

Fiber 1g

Sugar 2g

Cholesterol 0mg

Total Fat 1g

Protein 0g

Garden Wraps

Preparation Time: 20 minutes

Cooking Time: 10 minutes

Servings: 8

Ingredients:

1 cucumber, chopped

1 sweet corn

1 cabbage, shredded

1 tablespoon lettuce, minced

1 tomato, chopped

What you will need from the store cupboard:

3 tablespoons of rice vinegar

2 teaspoons peanut butter

1/3 cup onion paste

1/3 cup chili sauce

2 teaspoons of low-sodium soy sauce

Instructions:

Cut corn from the cob. Keep in a bowl.

Add the tomato, cabbage, cucumber, and onion paste. Now whisk the vinegar, peanut butter, and chili sauce together. Pour this over the vegetable mix. Toss for coating. Let this stand for 10 minutes. Take your slotted spoon and place ½ cup salad in every lettuce leaf. Fold the lettuce over your filling.

Nutrition:

Calories 64,

Carbohydrates 13g

Fiber 2g

Sugar 10g

Cholesterol 0mg

Total Fat 1g

Protein 2g

Stuffed Moroccan Mushrooms

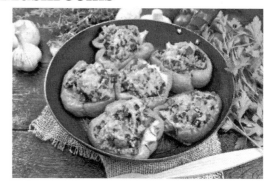

Preparation Time: 15 minutes

Cooking Time: 15 minutes

Servings: 12

Ingredients:

24 medium mushrooms

1/3 cup carrot, shredded

½ cup onion, chopped

½ teaspoon cumin, ground

¼ teaspoon coriander, ground

What you will need from the store cupboard:

1 garlic clove, minced

1 teaspoon of canola oil

¾ cup vegetable broth

½ teaspoon salt

Instructions:

Chop the mushroom stems finely. Keep the caps aside. Sauté the chopped stems, carrot and onion in your skillet in oil until they become tender and crisp. Now add the salt, garlic, coriander, and cumin. Cook while stirring for a minute. Add the broth and boil.

Remove from heat and keep aside for 5 minutes. Take a fork and fluff.

Place within the mushroom caps.

Keep on your baking sheet. Now bake for 5 minutes. The mushrooms should become tender.

Nutrition:

Calories 25,

Carbohydrates 5g

Fiber 1g

Sugar 1g

Cholesterol 0mg

Total Fat 0g

Protein 1g

Party Shrimp

Preparation Time: 15 minutes

Cooking Time: 10 minutes

Servings: 30

Ingredients:

16 oz. uncooked shrimp, peeled and deveined

1-1/2 teaspoons of juice from a lemon

½ teaspoon basil, chopped

1 teaspoon coriander, chopped

½ cup tomato

What you will need from the store cupboard:

1 tablespoon of olive oil

½ teaspoon Italian seasoning

½ teaspoon paprika

1 sliced garlic clove

1-1/2 teaspoons brown sugar

¼ teaspoon pepper

Instructions:

Bring together everything except the shrimp in a dish or bowl.

Add the shrimp.

Coat well by tossing. Set aside.

Drain the shrimp. Discard the marinade.

Keep them on a baking sheet. It should not be greased.

Broil each side for 4 minutes. The shrimp should become pink.

Nutrition:

Calories 14,

Carbohydrates 0g

Fiber 0g

Sugar 0g

Cholesterol 18mg

Total Fat 0g

Protein 2g

Zucchini Mini Pizzas

Preparation Time: 20 minutes

Cooking Time: 10 minutes

Servings: 24

Ingredients:

1 zucchini, cut into ¼ inch slices diagonally

½ cup pepperoni, small slices

1 teaspoon basil, minced

½ cup onion, chopped

1 cup tomatoes

What you will need from the store cupboard:

1/8 teaspoon pepper

1/8 teaspoon salt

3/4 cup mozzarella cheese, shredded

1/3 cup pizza sauce

Instructions:

Preheat your broiler.

Keep the zucchini in 1 layer on your greased baking sheet.

Add the onion and tomatoes.

Broil each side for 1 to 2 minutes till they become tender and crisp.

Now sprinkle pepper and salt.

Top with cheese, pepperoni, and sauce.

Broil for a minute. The cheese should melt.

Sprinkle basil on top.

Nutrition:

Calories 29,

Carbohydrates 1g

Fiber 0g

Sugar 1g

Cholesterol 5mg

Total Fat 2g

Protein 2g

Garlic-Sesame Pumpkin Seeds

Preparation Time: 10 minutes

Cooking Time: 20 minutes

Servings: 2

Ingredients:

1 egg white

1 teaspoon onion, minced

½ teaspoon caraway seeds

2 cups pumpkin seeds

1 teaspoon sesame seeds

What you will need from the store cupboard:

1 garlic clove, minced

1 tablespoon of canola oil

¾ teaspoon of kosher salt

Instructions:

Preheat your oven. Whisk together the oil and egg white in a bowl. Include pumpkin seeds. Coat well by tossing. Now stir in the onion, garlic, sesame seeds, caraway seeds, and salt.

Spread in 1 layer in your parchment-lined baking pan. Bake for 15 minutes until it turns golden brown.

Nutrition:

Calories 95,

Carbohydrates 9g

Fiber 3g

Sugar 0g

Cholesterol 0mg

Total Fat 5g

Protein 4g

Roasted Eggplant Spread

Preparation Time: 10 minutes

Cooking Time: 20 minutes

Servings: 2

Ingredients:

1 eggplant, medium, cut into small 1-inch pieces

2 red peppers, cut into 1-inch pieces

1 red onion, cut into 1-inch pieces

1 tablespoon tomato

4 toasted baguette slices

What you will need from the store cupboard:

3 garlic cloves, minced

3 tablespoons of olive oil

½ teaspoon pepper

½ teaspoon salt

Cooking spray

Instructions:

Preheat your oven.

Mix the olive oil, cloves, salt, and pepper. Keep vegetables in your bowl. Now toss with the oil mix. Transfer to your baking pan where you have applied cooking spray

Roast the vegetables till they get soft and are slightly brown. Now keep in a food processor.

Add the tomato and pulse until it blends. The mixture must be chunky.

Transfer to your bowl. Serve with the baguette.

Nutrition:

Calories 84,

Carbohydrates 9g

Fiber 3g

Sugar 5g

Cholesterol 0mg

Total Fat 5g

Protein 1g

Marinated Shrimp

Preparation Time: 10 minutes

Cooking Time: 20 minutes

Servings: 50

Ingredients:

30 oz. cooked shrimp, peeled and deveined

1 tablespoon parsley, minced

1/3 teaspoon dill weed

12 lime or lemon slices

½ cup red onion, sliced

What you will need from the store cupboard:

½ cup lime juice

½ cup canola oil

1/8 teaspoon of hot pepper sauce

½ teaspoon salt

Instructions:

Keep everything other than the shrimp in the bowl.

Now toss with the shrimp.

Set aside, stirring sometimes. Drain before you serve.

Nutrition:

Calories 28,

Carbohydrates 0g

Fiber 0g

Sugar 0g

Cholesterol 26mg

Total Fat 1g

Protein 3g

CHAPTER 15:

Dessert Recipes

Chocolate Pudding

Preparation time: 10 minutes

Cooking time: 20 minutes

Servings: 4

Ingredients:

2 tablespoons cocoa powder

2 tablespoons ghee, melted

2/3 cup heavy cream

2 tablespoons swerve

¼ teaspoon vanilla extract

Directions:

In a bowl, combine the cocoa with the ghee and the other ingredients whisk well and divide into 4 ramekins.

Bake at 350 degrees F for 20 minutes and serve warm.

Nutrition:

Calories 134

fat 14.4

fiber 0.4

carbs 3.4

protein 0.9

Coffee Cream

Preparation time: 10 minutes

Cooking time: 15 minutes

Servings: 4

Ingredients:

¼ cup brewed coffee

2 tablespoons swerve

2 cups heavy cream

1 teaspoon vanilla extract

2 tablespoons ghee, melted

2 eggs

Directions:

In a bowl, mix the coffee with the cream and the other ingredients, whisk well and divide into 4 ramekins and whisk well. Introduce the ramekins in the oven at 350 degrees F and bake for 15 minutes. Serve warm.

Nutrition:

Calories 304

fat 30.4

fiber 4 - carbs 4

protein 4

Walnut Balls

Preparation time: 10 minutes

Cooking time: 0 minutes

Servings: 6

Ingredients:

½ cup ghee, melted

4 tablespoons walnuts, chopped

1 tablespoon stevia

¼ cup coconut flesh, unsweetened and shredded

Directions:

In a bowl, combine the walnuts with the ghee and the other ingredients, stir well and spoon into round moulds.

Keep in the fridge until you serve them.

Nutrition:

Calories 194

fat 21.4

fiber 0.4

carbs 4

protein 1.4

Vanilla Cream

Preparation time: 10 minutes

Cooking time: 20 minutes

Servings: 4

Ingredients:

2 cups heavy cream

2 tablespoons stevia

1 teaspoon vanilla extract

1 cup heavy cream

2 eggs, whisked

1 teaspoon baking powder

Directions:

In a bowl, combine the cream with the stevia and the other ingredients and whisk well.

Divide into 4 ramekins, cook at 390 degrees F for 20 minutes, cool down and serve.

Nutrition:

Calories 344

fat 35.4

fiber 4

carbs 3.4

protein 4.6

Berry Cream

Preparation time: 10 minutes

Cooking time: 20 minutes

Servings: 4

Ingredients:

1 cup cream cheese

2 cups blackberries

1 tablespoon lime juice

1 tablespoon swerve

½ cup heavy cream

Directions:

In your blender, combine the blackberries with the cream and the other ingredients, pulse well and divide into 4 ramekins. Bake at 350 degrees F for 20 minutes, cool down and serve.

Nutrition:

Calories 284

fat 26.4

fiber 3.4

carbs 10.4

protein 5.7

Cream Cheese Ramekins

This special dessert will impress your loved ones for sure!

Preparation time: 10 minutes

Cooking time: 15 minutes

Servings: 6

Ingredients:

1 tablespoon vanilla extract

3 tablespoons ghee, melted

16 ounces cream cheese

½ cup swerve

1 teaspoon vanilla extract

Directions:

In a bowl, combine the vanilla with the ghee and the other ingredients, whisk well, divide into 6 ramekins, bake at 350 degrees F for 15 minutes, cool down and serve.

Nutrition:

Calories 324 - fat 32.4

fiber 4 - carbs 2.4 - protein 5.7

Avocado Cream

Preparation time: 10 minutes

Cooking time: 15 minutes

Servings: 4

Ingredients:

2 tablespoons avocado oil

8 ounces cream cheese

2 avocados, peeled, pitted and mashed

2 eggs, whisked

1 teaspoon baking powder

½ cup swerve

Directions:

In your blender, combine the cream cheese with the avocados and the other ingredients, pulse well, divide into 4 ramekins and bake at 360 degrees F for 15 minutes.

Cool the cream down and serve.

Nutrition:

Calories 314 - fat 29.4

fiber 3.4 - carbs 16.4

protein 8

Strawberry Stew

Preparation time: 10 minutes

Cooking time: 15 minutes

Servings: 4

Ingredients:

½ cup swerve

1-pound strawberries, halved

2 cups water

1 teaspoon vanilla extract

Directions:

In a pan, combine the strawberries with the swerve and the other ingredients, toss gently, bring to a simmer and cook over medium heat for 15 minutes.

Divide into bowls and serve cold.

Nutrition:

Calories 44

fat 4.4

fiber 2.4

carbs 3.4

protein 0.8

Coconut Muffins

Preparation time: 10 minutes

Cooking time: 25 minutes

Servings: 8

Ingredients:

½ cup ghee, melted

3 tablespoons swerve

1 cup coconut, unsweetened and shredded

¼ cup cocoa powder

2 eggs, whisked

¼ teaspoon vanilla extract

1 teaspoon baking powder

Directions:

In bowl, combine the ghee with the swerve, coconut and the other ingredients, stir well and divide into a lined muffin pan.

Bake at 370 degrees F for 25 minutes, cool down and serve.

Nutrition:

Calories 344

fat 35.4

fiber 3.4

carbs 8.4

protein 4.5

Blueberries Mousse

Preparation time: 10 minutes

Cooking time: 0 minutes

Servings: 6

Ingredients:

8 ounces heavy cream

1 teaspoon vanilla extract

1 tablespoon stevia

1 cup blueberries

Directions:

In a blender, combine the cream with the other ingredients, pulse well, divide into bowls and serve cold.

Nutrition:

Calories 214

fat 21.4

fiber 0.4

carbs 4

protein 1.4

Almond Berries Mix

Preparation time: 10 minutes

Cooking time: 12 minutes

Servings: 4

Ingredients:

1 cup almonds, chopped

1 cup strawberries

1 cup blackberries

¼ cup coconut milk

1 tablespoon stevia

Directions:

In a pan, combine the almonds with the strawberries and the other ingredients, bring to a simmer and cook over medium heat for 12 minutes.

Divide the mix into bowls and serve.

Nutrition:

Calories 264

fat 6.4 - fiber 4

carbs 4 - protein 6

Lime and Watermelon Mousse

Preparation time: 10 minutes

Cooking time: 0 minutes

Servings: 4

Ingredients:

1 cup heavy cream

1 tablespoon lime juice

1 tablespoon lime zest, grated

2 cups watermelon, peeled and cubed

1 cup cream cheese

Directions:

In a blender, combine the cream with the lime juice and the other ingredients, pulse well, divide into cups and serve cold.

Nutrition:

Calories 334

fat 31.4

fiber 0.4

carbs 9.4

protein 5.5

Eggs Cream

Preparation time: 2 hours

Cooking time: 10 minutes

Servings: 4

Ingredients:

4 eggs, whisked

¼ teaspoon vanilla extract

½ cup swerve

2 cups heavy cream

½ cup blackberries

Directions:

In a blender, combine the eggs with the vanilla and the other ingredients, pulse well, transfer to a pan, heat up over medium heat for 10 minutes, divide into bowls, cool down and keep in the fridge for 2 hours before serving.

Nutrition:

Calories 244 - fat 24

fiber 4 - carbs 6.4

protein 4

Chia Squares

Preparation time: 10 minutes

Cooking time: 20 minutes

Servings: 6

Ingredients:

1 cup ghee, melted

½ teaspoon baking powder

3 tablespoons chia seeds

2 tablespoons swerve

1 cup cream cheese

6 eggs, whisked

Directions:

In a bowl, combine the ghee with the chia seeds and the other ingredients, whisk well, pour everything into a square baking dish, introduce in the oven at 350 degrees F and bake for 20 minutes.

Cool down, slice into squares and serve.

Nutrition:

Calories 224

fat 4

fiber 0.4

carbs 4

protein 4

Plums Stew

Preparation time: 10 minutes

Cooking time: 20 minutes

Servings: 4

Ingredients:

1-pound plums, pitted and halved

2 cups water

2 teaspoons vanilla

1 tablespoon lime juice

5 tablespoons swerve

Directions:

In a pan, combine the plums with the water and the other ingredients, bring to a simmer and cook over medium heat for 20 minutes. Divide the mix into bowls and serve.

Nutrition:

Calories 174

fat 4.4 - fiber 4

carbs 4

protein 5

Plum Cream

Preparation time: 30 minutes

Cooking time: 0 minutes

Servings: 4

Ingredients:

1 tablespoon swerve

1 cup plums, pitted, peeled

1 teaspoon vanilla extract

2 cups heavy cream

Directions:

In a blender, combine the plums with the swerve and the other ingredients, pulse well, divide into bowls and keep in the fridge for 30 minutes before serving.

Nutrition:

Calories 144

fat 4

fiber 4

carbs 4

protein 4

Cold Berries and Plums Bowls

Preparation time: 5 minutes

Cooking time: 0 minutes

Servings: 4

Ingredients:

2 tablespoons swerve

1 cup plums, pitted and halved

1 teaspoon vanilla extract

1 cup blackberries

1 cup blueberries

2 tablespoons walnuts, chopped

Directions:

In a bowl, mix the plums with the blackberries and the other ingredients, toss and serve cold.

Nutrition:

Calories 404 - fat 24

fiber 4 - carbs 4

protein 7

Lime Avocado and Strawberries Mix

Preparation time: 5 minutes

Cooking time: 0 minutes

Servings: 4

Ingredients:

2 avocados, pitted, peeled and cubed

1 cup strawberries, halved

Juice of 1 lime

1 tablespoon stevia

Directions:

In a bowl, combine the avocados with the strawberries, lime juice and stevia, toss and serve cold.

Nutrition:

Calories 154

fat 4

fiber 4

carbs 4

protein 6

Avocado and Watermelon Salad

Preparation time: 2 hours

Cooking time: 0 minutes

Servings: 4

Ingredients:

2 avocados pitted, peeled and cubed

2 cups watermelon, peeled and cubed

1 tablespoon stevia

1 cup heavy cream

1 tablespoon mint, chopped

Directions:

In a bowl, combine the avocados with the watermelon and the other ingredients, toss and keep in the fridge for 2 hours before serving.

Nutrition:

Calories 274

fat 24.4

fiber 6.4

carbs 14.4

protein 2.8

Coconut Raspberries Mix

Preparation time: 10 minutes

Cooking time: 15 minutes

Servings: 4

Ingredients:

1 cup coconut milk

2 tablespoons coconut flesh, unsweetened and shredded

1 cup raspberries

3 tablespoons swerve

½ teaspoon vanilla extract

Directions:

In a blender, combine the coconut with the raspberries and the other ingredients, pulse well, divide into 4 ramekins, introduce in the oven at 360 degrees F for 15 minutes, cool down and serve.

Nutrition:

Calories 394 - fat 37.4

fiber 9.4 - carbs 16.4 - protein 4.2

Cinnamon Cream

Preparation time: 2 hours

Cooking time: 10 minutes

Servings: 4

Ingredients:

2 tablespoons swerve

1 cup coconut milk

1 cup heavy cream

1 tablespoon cinnamon powder

¼ teaspoon ginger, ground

Directions:

In a bowl, combine the cream with the milk and the other ingredients, whisk well, transfer to a pot, heat up over medium heat for 10 minutes and divide into bowls. Keep in the fridge for 2 hours before serving.

Nutrition:

Calories 244 - fat 25.4

fiber 1.4

carbs 5.4

protein 2

Chocolate Cookies

Preparation time: 10 minutes

Cooking time: 20 minutes

Servings: 6

Ingredients:

2 cups walnuts, chopped

2 eggs, whisked

¼ cup avocado oil

2 tablespoons swerve

¼ cup cocoa powder

1 teaspoon baking powder

Directions:

In your food processor, combine the walnuts with the eggs and the other ingredients, pulse well, scoop tablespoons out of this mix, put them on a lined baking sheet, flatten them a bit and cook at 360 degrees F for 20 minutes.

Serve the cookies cold.

Nutrition:

Calories 454

fat 41.4

fiber 6.4 - carbs 11.4

protein 19

Special Dessert

Preparation time: 10 minutes

Cooking time: 0 minutes

Servings: 6

Ingredients:

1 cup blueberries

1 cup almonds, chopped

½ cup walnuts, chopped

1 cup blackberries

1 tablespoon swerve

1 tablespoon coconut oil, melted

Directions:

In a bowl, combine the berries with the almonds, and the other ingredients, toss and serve cold.

Nutrition:

Calories 224 - fat 34

fiber 4 - carbs 4 - protein 6

Coconut and Mint Cookies

Preparation time: 10 minutes

Cooking time: 15 minutes

Servings: 6

Ingredients:

1 cup almond flour

1 cup coconut, unsweetened and shredded

2 eggs, whisked

½ cup coconut cream

½ cup coconut oil, melted

3 tablespoons swerve

2 teaspoons mint, dried

2 teaspoons baking powder

Directions:

In a bowl, mix the almond flour with the coconut and the other ingredients, and stir well.

Shape balls out of this mix, place them on a lined baking sheet, flatten them, introduce in the oven at 370 degrees F and bake for 15 minutes.

Serve them cold.

Nutrition:

Calories 194 - fat 7.34

fiber 2.4 - carbs 4 - protein 3

Avocado Bars

Preparation time: 10 minutes

Cooking time: 30 minutes

Servings: 6

Ingredients:

1 teaspoon vanilla extract

½ cup ghee, melted

2 tablespoons swerve

1 avocado, peeled, pitted and mashed

2 cups almond flour

1 tablespoon cocoa powder

Directions:

In a bowl, mix the ghee with the vanilla and the other ingredients and stir everything.

Transfer this to baking pan, spread evenly on the bottom, introduce in the oven at 350 degrees F and bake for 30 minutes.

Cool down, cut into bars and serve.

Nutrition:

Calories 234

fat 12.4

fiber 4.4

carbs 5.4

protein 5.8

Orange Cake

Preparation time: 10 minutes

Cooking time: 20 minutes

Servings: 12

Ingredients:

6 eggs

1 orange, cut in quarters

1 teaspoon vanilla extract

1 teaspoon baking powder

9 ounces almond meal

4 tablespoons swerve

A pinch of salt

2 tablespoons orange zest

2 ounces stevia

4 ounces cream cheese

4 ounces coconut yogurt

Directions:

In your food processor, pulse orange very well.

Add almond meal, swerve, eggs, baking powder, vanilla extract and a pinch of salt and pulse well again.

Transfer this into 2 spring form pans, introduce in the oven at 350 degrees F and bake for 20 minutes.

Meanwhile, in a bowl, mix cream cheese with orange zest, coconut yogurt and stevia and stir well.

Place one cake layer on a plate, add half of the cream cheese mix, add the other cake layer and top with the rest of the cream cheese mix.

Spread it well, slice and serve.

Enjoy!

Nutrition:

Calories 204

fat 14

fiber 4

carbs 4

protein 8

Tasty Nutella

Preparation time: 10 minutes

Cooking time: 0 minutes

Servings: 6

Ingredients:

2 ounces coconut oil

4 tablespoons cocoa powder

1 teaspoon vanilla extract

1 cup walnuts, halved

4 tablespoons stevia

Directions:

In your food processor, mix cocoa powder with oil, vanilla, walnuts and stevia and blend very well. Keep in the fridge for a couple of hours and then serve.

Enjoy!

Nutrition:

Calories 104

fat 14

fiber 4

carbs 4

protein 2

Mug Cake

Preparation time: 2 minutes

Cooking time: 3 minutes

Servings: 1

Ingredients:

4 tablespoons almond meal

2 tablespoon ghee

1 teaspoon stevia

1 tablespoon cocoa powder, unsweetened

1 egg

1 tablespoon coconut flour

¼ teaspoon vanilla extract

½ teaspoon baking powder

Directions:

Put the ghee in a mug and introduce in the microwave for a couple of seconds.

Add cocoa powder, stevia, egg, baking powder, vanilla and coconut flour and stir well.

Add almond meal as well, stir again, introduce in the microwave and cook for 2 minutes.

Serve your mug cake with berries on top.

Enjoy!

Nutrition:

Calories 454

fat 34

fiber 4

carbs 14

protein 20

Delicious Sweet Buns

Preparation time: 10 minutes

Cooking time: 30 minutes

Servings: 8

Ingredients:

½ cup coconut flour

1/3 cup psyllium husks

2 tablespoons swerve

1 teaspoon baking powder

A pinch of salt

½ teaspoon cinnamon

½ teaspoon cloves, ground

4 eggs

Some chocolate chips, unsweetened

1 cup hot water

Directions:

In a bowl, mix flour with psyllium husks, swerve, baking powder, salt, cinnamon, cloves and chocolate chips and stir well. Add water and egg, stir well until you obtain a dough, shape 8 buns and arrange them on a lined baking sheet. Introduce in the oven at 350 degrees and bake for 30 minutes. Serve these buns with some almond milk and enjoy!

Nutrition:

Calories 104 - fat 4

fiber 4 - carbs 4

protein 6

Lemon Custard

Preparation time: 10 minutes

Cooking time: 30 minutes

Servings: 6

Ingredients:

1- and 1/3-pint almond milk

4 tablespoons lemon zest

4 eggs

5 tablespoons swerve

2 tablespoons lemon juice

Directions:

In a bowl, mix eggs with milk and swerve and stir very well.

Add lemon zest and lemon juice, whisk well, pour into ramekins and place them into a baking dish with some water on the bottom.

Bake in the oven at 360 degrees F for 30 minutes.

Leave custard to cool down before serving it.

Enjoy!

Nutrition:

Calories 124

fat 4

fiber 4

carbs 4

protein 7

Conclusion

By some accounts, half of all Americans have been diagnosed with either diabetes or prediabetes. Learning to cook and plan meals that fit with a diabetes meal plan will help you and your loved ones live longer, healthier lives.

The two components of any healthy lifestyle are diet and exercise. Alongside physical activity, reducing the sugars in your diet can help your blood sugars remain stable. This cookbook makes a great complement to your regular exercise program. Many of these recipes can be prepared in large batches on the weekend for easy meals throughout the workweek.

Why wait? You can make many of the recipes in this cookbook without specialty ingredients or equipment.

Today is the best time to take control of your diet and your health!

By taking the time to learn to cook your favorite recipes in a diabetes-friendly way and evaluating which sugars your body absorbs most slowly, you can find increased energy and health. Using the recipes from this cookbook, your entire family can enjoy tasty, delicious meals and snacks while you keep your diabetes under control.

Made in the USA
Las Vegas, NV
05 December 2020